Optimum Men's Health

An In-Depth Guide to Men's Health Issues
Including Prevention and Treatment Options

By Jon Shelton

Copyrights and Trademarks

Disclaimer and Legal Notice

Foreword

How many times do you go to the doctor in any given year? Do you keep up with your routine screenings and vaccinations? Do you know what your cholesterol level is? Your blood pressure? Your BMI?

If you didn't answer "Yes" to any of these questions, then you may want to seriously reconsider. Many men underestimate the importance of annual physicals and routine screenings, not realizing that these very simple things could make the difference between catching a serious disease in the early stages and dying from it.

Your health is not something you should be taking for granted – you can lose it in an instant. The purpose of this book is to educate you about common men's health issues and to teach you the importance of keeping up with routine checkups, screenings, and vaccinations. Preventive medicine is not complicated (it doesn't even have to be time-consuming) but it can make a big difference. Don't you want to live the longest, healthiest life you can?

So, if you are ready to take responsibility for yourself and your health, simply turn the page and keep reading!

Table of Contents

Introduction

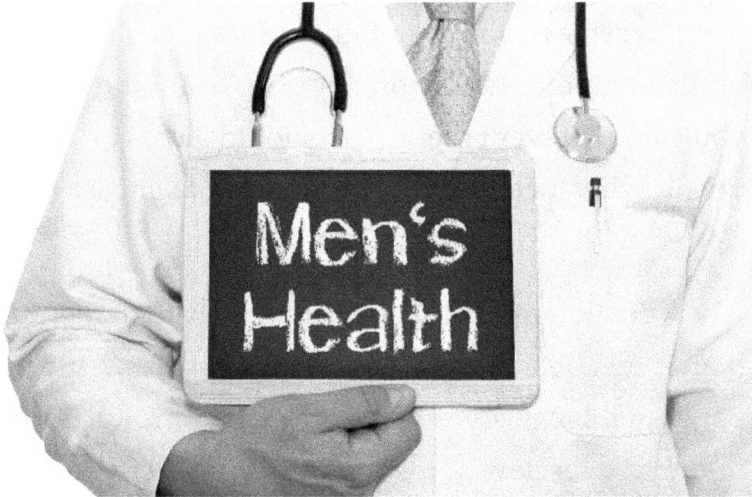

Did you know that men live an average of 5 years shorter than women and that they die at higher rates from the top 10 causes of death than women? According to the Men's Health Network, men are thought to have weaker immune systems than men and approximately 75% of suicides each year are committed by men. But are men really the "weaker sex" or are they simply troubled by different health issues than women?

Studies have shown that women are much more likely to keep up with their annual physical exam and routine preventive health screenings than men. This means that they are more likely to catch serious health problems in the early stages when they are still treatable. As a man, you need to take responsibility for your health and that means educating yourself about the top men's health issues. If you want to achieve and maintain optimum health, you need to understand the risk factors for disease and do everything you can to prevent them. You should also work with your doctor when health problems do arise to ensure that you get started with the proper treatment.

If you are curious to learn more about men's health issues, this book is the perfect place to start. Within the pages of this book you will receive an introduction to and an in-depth overview of the top men's health issues as well as important information about preventive health screenings. You will also receive detailed information about the top men's health issues in key categories such as cardiovascular health, digestive health, mental health, and more. By the time you finish this book you will have a deeper understanding of what the top men's health issues are and how to prevent them.

So, if you are ready to learn how to achieve and maintain optimum men's health, just turn the page and keep reading!

Useful Terms to Know

Acute Care – Care that is generally provided for a short period of time to treat a new illness or a flare-up from an existing condition.

Acute Disease – A disease characterized by a single or repeated episode of relatively rapid onset and short duration.

After-Care – Care provided to patients after their release from institutional care.

Agent – A factor (such as a microorganism) which is essential for the occurrence of a disease.

Assistive Device – Equipment that enables an individual who requires assistance to perform the daily activities essential to maintain health and autonomy.

Caregiver – A person who provides support and assistance with various activities to persons with disabilities or long-term conditions.

Cause of Death – The underlying condition to which death is attributed.

Chronic Condition – A disease which has one or more of the following characteristics: is permanent, leaves residual disability, is caused by non-reversible pathological alternation, or may be expected to require a long period of supervision or care.

Clinic – A facility devoted to diagnosis and treatment or rehabilitation of outpatients.

Copayment – Or copay; the specified portion that health insurance may require a person to pay toward medical bills or services.

Diagnosis – The process of determining health status and the factors responsible for producing it.

Disability – A restriction or lack of ability to perform an activity in the manner considered to be normal.

Disease – A failure of the adaptive mechanisms of an organism to counteract adequately to stimuli and stresses which results in a disturbance of the function or structure of some part; an illness.

Efficacy – The extent to which a specific procedure or service produces a beneficial result.

Emergency – A sudden unexpected onset of illness or injury which requires immediate care.

Episode – The period in which a health problem or illness exists, from its outset to its resolution.

Health – The state of complete physical, mental, and social well-being, not merely the absence of disease or infirmity.

Illness – A person's own perceptions, experience, and evaluation of a disease or condition.

Incontinence – Loss of bladder and/or bowel control.

Inpatient – An individual who has been admitted to a hospital or facility for diagnosis and/or treatment that requires at least one overnight stay.

Life Expectancy – The average number of years of life remaining to a person at a particular age based on age-specific death rates.

Mental Health – The absence of psychiatric disorders/traits.

Mental Illness – Forms of illness in which psychological, emotional or behavioral disturbances are dominant.

Mortality – Death; used to describe the relation of deaths to the population in which they occur.

Outpatient – A patient who is receiving ambulatory care at a hospital or other facility without being admitted.

Patient – A person in contact with the health system seeking attention for a health condition.

Physician – A professional person qualified by education and authorized by law to practice medicine.

Pre-Existing Condition – A condition developed prior to applying for a health insurance policy.

Prevention – Aimed at promoting health, preserving health, and restoring health when it is impaired and to minimize suffering and distress.

Preventive Care – Care that has the aim of preventing disease or its consequences.

Primary Care Physician – A patient's regular doctor.

Screening – The use of procedures and measures to identify and differentiate well persons who have a disease or condition or a high risk from those who probably do not.

Self-Care – Health activities, including promotion, maintenance, treatment, care, and health related decision-making, carried out by individuals and families.

Side Effect – An effect, other than the intended one, produced by a procedure or regimen.

Specialist – A health professional who is specially trained in a certain branch of his or her profession related to specific services or procedures.

Symptom – A sign or indication of a disorder or disease.

Treatment - A process designed to achieve a desired health status for a patient.

Chapter One: Understanding the Top Men's Health Issues

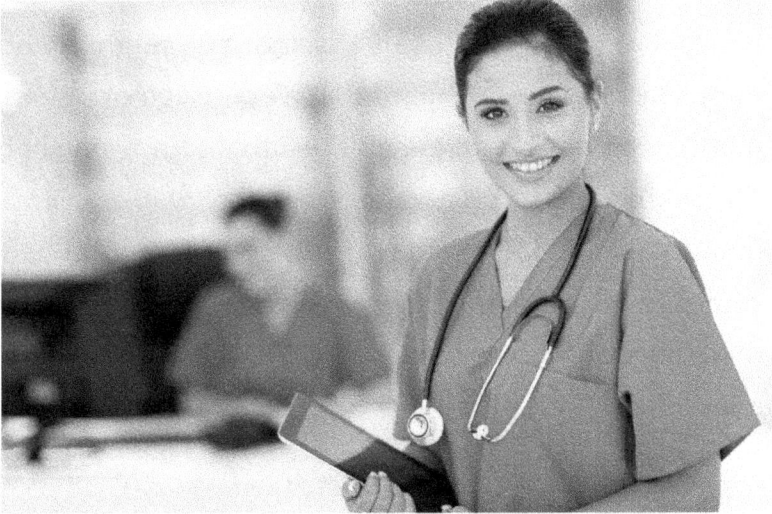

If you hate going to the doctor, you are not alone –
many men neglect their annual checkup, not realizing that it
could have a serious impact on their health. In this chapter
you will learn about the importance of an annual physical
and you will receive an introduction to some of the most
common men's health issues. The information in this chapter
will serve as an introduction for the rest of the book in which
these issues will be discussed in depth.

1.) Men's Health Statistics

If you were to open up a conversation about the differences between men and women, there are certain topics that you would likely discuss. You might mention things like the wage gap, or the average age of puberty – you might even talk about general health and hygiene habits. These kinds of differences between the two sexes are quantifiable and they are worthy of discussion. When it comes to the differences between men and women, however, these may not be the biggest differences that should be given attention.

Many men do not realize that there are some significant differences between men and women when it comes to issues related to health and longevity. <u>If you do just a little bit of research, however, you will come across some shocking statistics such as the following</u>:

- Men are 24% less likely than women to have visited their doctor within the past 12 months.
- Men are 22% more likely than women to have neglected routine cholesterol tests.
- Men have a 28% higher risk for being hospitalized for congestive heart failure and 32% more likely to be hospitalized for the long-term complications of diabetes.

- Men are twice as likely as women to have a leg or foot amputated due to complications of diabetes.
- Men are 24% more likely than women to be hospitalized for pneumonia that could have easily been prevented by getting a vaccination.

What you may notice if you take the time to carefully review this list of statistics, is that many of the problems mentioned are easily preventable. You may notice a theme – that men tend to be more likely than women to neglect simple health checks or vaccinations which could prevent a serious health problem from occurring later on down the road. This may not be true for all men, but it certainly does seem to be a common issue.

According to the Social Security Administration, men who reach the age of 65 can be expected to live an average of 2.3 years less than women who reach the age of 65. A study of human life expectancy during the last decade of the 20th century taken by Bertrand Desjardins, a researcher at the University of Montreal, notes that U.S. male life expectancy was an average of 6.7 years shorter on the whole. Desjardins also notes that the mortality of males is higher than that of females from the very beginning of their lives – as much as 25% to 30% higher!

But what exactly should you take away from these statistics? These statistics may be saddening – scary, even –

but they may be just the kind of reality check you need to start taking your own health and wellness more seriously. As a man, you are already disadvantaged in terms of life expectancy and mortality – don't you want to do what you can to reduce your health risks and to live the longest, healthiest life you can?

If you are serious about taking your health more seriously, it all starts with a visit to your primary care physician. A yearly checkup or annual physical is a must for both men and women. During this checkup your doctor will make note of certain things like your height, weight, and body mass index (BMI) - he may also order various tests or health screenings. The information gathered from these tests will help your doctor to determine whether you have any health problems that need to be addressed.

Many men neglect to schedule annual physicals when they are not feeling physically ill. You must realize, however, that preventive care is extremely important – catching a disease in the early stages could drastically improve your chances of making a full recovery. Furthermore, keeping up to date with your immunizations could completely protect you from certain illnesses which have the potential to be very serious. An annual physical takes just a few minutes to schedule an generally no more than an hour to complete – isn't your health worth an hour of your time?

If you can't be convinced to schedule an annual physical each year, here is a list of reasons that may indicate the need for a checkup:

- You are sick or have been exposed to some kind of illness.
- You are displaying symptoms of an illness or have experienced changes that concern you.
- You have a chronic or ongoing condition that needs to be managed.
- You want to check in about side effects and dosage for any medication you may be taking.
- You have certain bad habits that could affect your health such as drinking, smoking, or overeating.
- You have a family history of certain diseases, especially serious diseases.

These reasons are all valid when it comes to motivation for scheduling an annual physical. If you can't be convinced by the potential benefits of preventive care for your own health, think about the benefits it could have for your wallet. If you have health insurance, the cost of your annual exam is probably completely covered except for any applicable copay. The cost of ignoring a potential problem, however, could be very high – you may end up going to the emergency room for treatment and, if the condition is allowed to progress, you may even need to be hospitalized. Medical expenses add up quickly and, in many cases, they can be prevented by catching a problem early during a simple yearly checkup.

By now the benefits of an annual checkup should be obvious to you. In the next section you will receive an overview of common men's health issues that your doctor may look for during your annual exam. You will also receive a list of recommended health screenings for men determined by age.

2.) What are the Most Common Men's Health Issues?

Many men think that they are invincible – as long as they feel okay for the most part, they do not see any reason to go to the doctor, even for an annual checkup. What many of these men do not realize is that serious health problems can be lurking just beneath the surface and you may not experience any outward symptoms until the disease has progressed. Some of the most dangerous silent killers include various types of cancer and heart disease. In this section you will find an overview of some of the most common men's health issues.

- **Heart Disease** – According to the Centers for Disease Control (CDC), one in four men has some form of heart disease – furthermore, heart disease is the number one killer of both men and women. In fact, heart disease can begin to manifest 10 years earlier in men than women.

- **Stroke** – The third most common cause of death in the United States, stroke affects more than 3 million men each year. High blood pressure is extremely common in men under the age of 45 and it greatly increases your risk for stroke.

- **Cancer** – In all of its many forms, cancer is the second leading cause of death in the United States. Lung cancer is the most common type of cancer, taking more lives than colon, prostate, and breast cancers combined. In men, the most common form of cancer is prostate cancer and it is the second leading type of cancer death in men, after lung cancer.

- **Depression/Suicide** – According to the National Institute of Mental Health (NIMH), more than 6 million men suffer from depression each year. It is also worth noting that men are four times as likely as women to commit suicide. The NIMH also notes that this may be partially due to the fact that depression is largely underdiagnosed in men as compared to women.

- **Respiratory Disease** – Emphysema, COPD, and lung cancer (among other forms of respiratory disease) can easily become life-threatening. According to the

American Lung Association, each year more men are diagnosed with lung cancer than in the previous year.

- **Alcoholism** – The Centers for Disease Control suggest that men tend to binge drink twice as much as women and they face much higher rates of alcohol-related deaths and hospitalizations as well. Excessive alcohol consumption increases the risk for various cancers and it can interfere with hormone production and testicular function.

- **Accidents/Injuries** – Not only are men more likely than women to skip their annual checkups, but they are also more likely to put themselves in potentially dangerous situations. The CDC notes that motor vehicle death rates were twice as high for male drivers and passengers than for females. In fact, unintentional injury was the leading cause of death for men in 2006.

- **Liver Disease** – The liver is responsible for ridding the body of toxic substances and its function can be impaired by a number of serious diseases such as cirrhosis, viral hepatitis, liver cancer, or alcoholic liver disease. Alcohol and tobacco use can increase your risk for developing liver disease.

- **Diabetes** – You may not think of diabetes as a life-threatening disease, but it can become very dangerous if neglected or if not properly managed. Untreated diabetes often leads to nerve and kidney damage as well as vision problems and an increased risk for heart attack and stroke.

- **Influenza/Pneumonia** – Like diabetes, influenza and pneumonia may not seem particularly dangerous but men are 25% more likely than women to die from these diseases. In fact, influenza and pneumococcal infection are two of the leading health risks for men – these risks increase in men who have diabetes, AIDS, cancer or compromised immune systems due to other factors.

- **HIV/AIDS** – According to a 2010 study conducted by the CDC, men account for 76% of people infected with HIV. Furthermore, men who choose to have sex with men account for most of the new and existing HIV infections in the United States.

These are just some of the many health issues known to affect men. In the next section you will receive a list of recommended health screenings for men of certain ages. Keeping up with your routine health screenings will help to reduce your risk for these and other diseases.

3.) Recommended Health Screenings by Age

The symptoms for certain illnesses are obvious and undeniable. For example, if you have the flu you will probably develop a fever, cough, and chills. There are some diseases, however, which can develop silently and slowly. The best way to protect yourself from disease is to keep up with your annual physicals and to get routine screenings as recommended by your doctor. A screening is simply a test that looks for a disease before you show any symptoms. For example, a blood cholesterol test checks for high LDL ("bad" cholesterol) levels.

Below you will find a list of the top men's health screening as well as the age most doctors recommend them:

- **Abdominal Aortic Aneurysm** – An AAA is a bulging in the abdominal aorta, the largest artery in the body, and it can burst and cause bleeding and death. You should get an AAA test if you are between the ages of 65 and 75, especially if you have ever been a smoker.

- **Colon Cancer** – This test is recommended annually for all men starting at the age of 50. If you have a family history of colorectal cancer, you may need to start getting screened earlier.

- **Depression** – If you have experienced feelings of sadness or hopelessness or if you have lost interest or pleasure in things you once enjoyed, you may need a depression screening.

- **Diabetes** – If you have high blood pressure or if you take medication for your blood pressure, a diabetes screening is highly recommended.

- **Hepatitis C** – All men should be screened for this disease once if they were born between 1945 and 1965, if they have ever injected drugs, and if you received a blood transfusion prior to 1992.

- **High Blood Cholesterol** – Men over the age of 35 should have their blood cholesterol checked regularly. High blood pressure can greatly increase your risk for heart disease and stroke. Factors that increase your risk further include tobacco use, overweight/obesity, diabetes, high blood pressure, and family history of heart disease.

- **High Blood Pressure** – All men should have their blood pressure checked at least every 2 years.
- **HIV** – Men who are 65 or younger should be screened for HIV.

- **Lung Cancer** – One of the leading causes of death in men, lung cancer screenings are recommended between the ages of 55 and 80. If you have a 30 pack-year smoking history, if you currently smoke, or if you quit smoking with the past 15 years, your risk is higher.

- **Overweight/Obesity** – Even if you track your weight at home, you should have your BMI measured by a doctor at least once per year. A healthy BMI is between 18.5 and 25 while a BMI of 30 or higher indicates obesity.

In addition to getting these recommended health screenings, your doctor may also recommend the use of certain preventive medications. For example, taking aspirin on a daily basis may help to prevent heart attacks in men aged 45 and older. You should also stay up to date with your immunizations.

Chapter Two: Men's Heart Health

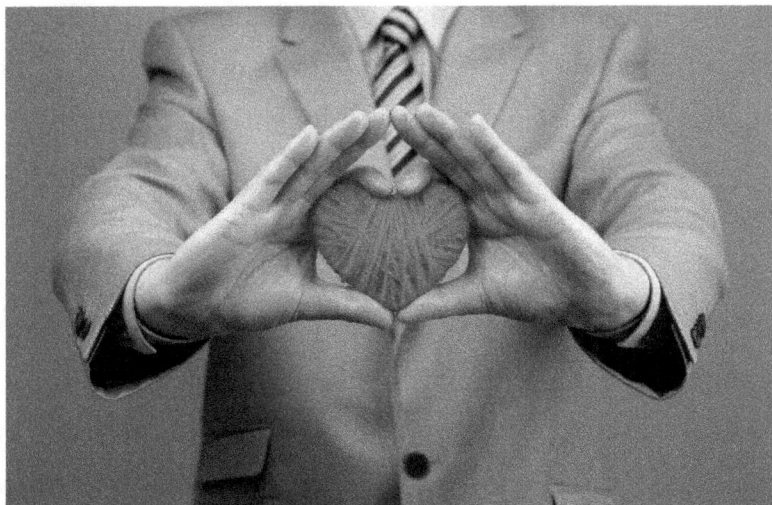

When you think of cardiac health issues you probably think of heart disease. What you may not realize is that cardiovascular disease comes in a variety of different forms and some are more dangerous than others. Your heart is an extremely important organ – it is responsible for pumping your life's blood throughout your body, supplying oxygen and nutrients to your vital organs. Cardiac health is not something you should take for granted! In this chapter you will learn the basics about common cardiac health issues affecting men as well as tips for maintaining good heart health.

1.) Overview of the Cardiovascular System

The cardiovascular system is responsible for pumping blood throughout the body. It consists of the heart (the organ which does the pumping) and its various conduits – capillaries, veins, and arteries. The blood carries various nutrients and wastes as well as oxygen and immune cells that play a role in supporting the basic function of other cells and organs in the body. Arteries are the blood vessels that move blood away from the heart while veins are the vessels that transport it back toward the heart. Capillaries carry blood to the tissue cells where gases, wastes, and nutrients can be exchanged.

The human body usually has a blood volume of 5 liters (a little more than one gallon) and the total blood volume generally passes through the heart once each minute. The heart usually pumps blood at a specific rate which is called cardiac output (CO). Cardiac output does vary, however, with the demands of the body and it can be influenced by various other factors. A normal heart rate is about 72 beats per minute which makes the average cardiac cycle about 0.8 seconds long.

In terms of anatomy, the cardiovascular system consists of two primary components: the heart and the blood vessels. There are also two specific circuits through which blood flows. The pulmonary circuit is the path blood takes when flowing through the lungs. The systemic circuit is the path of blood as it flows through the rest of the human body. As the heart contracts, it generates blood pressure in the arteries which helps to move the blood along and various one-way valves in the heart and veins make sure that the blood only flows one direction.

The human heart is composed of four chambers: the left and right atria, and the left and right ventricles. The right atrium receives oxygen-poor blood from throughout the body and pumps it into the right ventricle which then pumps the blood into the lungs for oxygenation. The left atrium receives the newly oxygenated blood from the lungs and pumps it into the left ventricle which then pumps it throughout the body as needed. In addition to these chambers, two other important structures are the pericardium – the membranous sac that surrounds the heart – and the myocardium – the cardiac muscle tissue which contracts in order to pump blood.

2.) The Top Men's Cardiac Health Issues

According to the American Heart Association (AHA), more than one in three adult men has some kind of cardiovascular disease. Furthermore, males represented nearly 50% of deaths from cardiovascular disease in 2009.

While cardiovascular disease (CVD) is one of the most common cardiac health issues affecting men, there are several others which include:

- Coronary Heart Disease (CHD)
- Angina Pectoris
- Congenital Cardiovascular Defects
- Stroke
- High Blood Pressure (HBP)
- Heart Failure (HF)
- High Blood Cholesterol

In the following pages you will receive an overview of each of these conditions including their symptoms and risk factors. The more you know about cardiovascular disease, the better you can protect yourself against it.

a.) Coronary Heart Disease (CHD)

This disease occurs when a waxy substance known as plaque begins to build up in the coronary arteries over a period of many years, leading to a condition known as atherosclerosis. In time, this buildup of plaque has the potential to harden, forming an obstruction that narrows the coronary artery and reduces blood flow to the heart. The plaque formation could also rupture, or break open, causing a blood clot to form which could also lead to an obstruction of blood flow.

When blood flow to the heart is impaired, it can lead to angina (chest pain or discomfort) or even a heart attack. If blood flow isn't restored, the heart muscle can actually begin to die. Over time, untreated CHD can lead to heart failure or to arrhythmias, abnormal heart beat. Treatment for CHD may involve prescription medication as well as lifestyle changes. In some cases, surgery may even be required to correct the problem.

b.) Angina Pectoris

Also known as stable angina, angina pectoris is the medical term for chest pain related to coronary heart disease. This condition develops when the heart doesn't receive enough oxygenated blood, usually because one or more of the coronary arteries has been blocked. Symptoms of angina generally include uncomfortable pressure or fullness in the chest, or a squeezing pain in the center of the chest. You may also feel pain or discomfort in your neck, jaw, shoulder, back, or arm.

c.) Congenital Cardiovascular Defects

Congenital heart defects are a problem with the structure of the heart that is present at birth. These defects may affect the interior walls of the heart, the valves inside the heart, or the veins and arteries that carry blood to the heart or from the heart to the rest of the body. In many cases, congenital heart defects change the normal blood flow coming from the heart and symptoms can range in severity from mild to life-threatening.

Many congenital heart defects are simple enough that they need no treatment or that they are easily repaired. For people with complex heart defects, however, lifelong treatment may be required. According to the National Heart, Lung, and Blood Institute, about 1 million American adults are living with congenital heart defects – some of the most common kinds include septal defects (holes in the heart), patent ductus arteriosus, and narrowed valves. The most common complex heart defect is called tetralogy of Fallot and it is a combination of the following four defects:

- Pulmonary valve stenosis
- An enlarged VSD
- An overriding aorta
- Right ventricular hypertrophy

Treatment for congenital heart defects vary depending on the type and severity of the defect. Repairs can frequently be made with various catheter procedures, though some may require surgery.

d.) Stroke

A stroke occurs when blood flow to the brain is cut off and, when that happens, the brain cells are deprived of oxygen and they begin to die off. The most common symptoms of stroke include numbness or weakness on one side of the body which may be accompanied by confusion, difficulty speaking, loss of coordination, changes in vision, or an intense headache. These symptoms can come on suddenly and without warning. If blood flow is not restored quickly, you could die.

There are technically two kinds of stroke – hemorrhagic stroke and ischemic stroke. Hemorrhagic stroke occurs when a brain aneurysm bursts or a weakened blood vessel begins to leak. An ischemic stroke occurs when a blood vessel that supplies blood to the brain becomes blocked by a blood clot. There is also something called a transient ischemic attack (TIA) which mimics the symptoms of stroke and it occurs when blood flow to part of the brain is cut off for a short period of time.

e.) High Blood Pressure (HBP)

Also known as hypertension, high blood pressure is a common condition in which the force of blood against the artery walls (your blood pressure) becomes high enough that it could cause heart problems such as cardiovascular disease. Your blood pressure is measured according to the amount of blood being pumped out by your heart as well as the amount of resistance to blood flow in your arteries. The more blood your heart pumps, the more narrowed your arteries become and the higher your blood pressure rises.

In many cases, high blood pressure doesn't cause any negative symptoms for several years. Even if you don't have symptoms, however, you could be sustaining damage to your blood vessels. Uncontrolled hypertension significantly increases your risk for heart attack and stroke. Fortunately, high blood pressure is easy to detect and it is fairly easy to control as well. Making healthy changes to your diet and lifestyle can help you to manage your blood pressure, as can prescription medications.

f.) Heart Failure (HF)

Sometimes known as congestive heart failure, heart failure occurs when your heart muscle doesn't pump blood as efficiently as it should. There are various conditions which can lead to congestive heart failure including coronary artery disease (narrowed arteries) or even high blood pressure. Over time, these conditions can weaken your heart to the point that it is no longer able to pump blood as well as it should or it could make your heart too stiff to fill properly with blood.

Some of the conditions that lead to heart failure cannot be reversed, but there are treatments available to help you managed the symptoms and increase your longevity. Healthy lifestyle changes, for example, can improve your heart health as well as your quality of life in general. You should also make sure that other chronic conditions like diabetes, high blood pressure, obesity, and coronary artery disease are kept under control. There are also medications which can help treat heart failure.

g.) High Blood Cholesterol

Cholesterol is a fat-like substance that is present in your blood and, when there is too much of it, it can build up in the walls of your arteries. Over time, this accumulation can cause your arteries to become narrowed which can slow

or block blood flow to the heart. High blood pressure itself
does not cause any observable symptoms so it is important
to have your cholesterol tested regularly to detect high blood
pressure before it becomes a problem. Individuals over the
age of 20 should have their cholesterol tested at least every 5
years.

3.) Tips for Improving Cardiovascular Health

Your cardiovascular health is not something you
should take for granted because even minor heart issues can
lead to big problems. Fortunately, improving and
maintaining good heart health is not difficult – it may,
however, require a certain degree of intentionality and time.
Here are a few simple tips men can use to improve and
maintain cardiovascular health:

- **Watch your sodium intake**. Excess sodium intake can
  damage your blood vessels and increase your risk for
  developing hypertension which, in turn, increases your
  risk for various forms of heart disease. The American
  Heart Association recommends a daily sodium intake
  around 1,500 mg.

- **Get regular exercise**. You shouldn't be surprised to
  learn that regular exercise is one of the best things you

can do to improve and maintain heart health. As little as 30 minutes of aerobic exercise five times a week can significantly reduce your risk for heart disease.

- **Maintain a healthy weight**. Overweight and obesity increases your risk for a number of chronic diseases including heart disease. The more weight you are carrying around, the harder your heart has to work and the more likely you are to develop problems. Following a healthy diet and getting some regular exercise can help you to achieve and maintain a healthy bodyweight which, in turn, will reduce your risk for heart disease.

- **Quit smoking as soon as possible**. According to the American Heart Association, quitting smoking can reduce your risk for heart disease as much as (or more than) taking prescription medications designed for that purpose.

- **Get plenty of sleep**. Getting enough sleep has a serious impact on your health in general but it is particularly beneficial for your heart health. Aim for at least 7 hours a night for the maximum benefit and try to stick to a regular sleep schedule, if you can manage.

- **Watch your fat intake**. Contrary to popular belief, all fats are not bad. It is true that you want to avoid saturated fats and trans fats (the kinds that come from fried and processed foods) but monounsaturated fats and omega fatty acids are very good for your body, particularly your heart.

- **Follow a healthy diet**. You have probably heard the saying "you are what you eat" – this simply means that the food you eat has a direct impact on your health. A clean diet of wholesome foods will give your heart the energy it needs to maintain proper function without having to waste extra energy digesting processed foods.

- **Manage your stress level**. Chronic stress is a very serious (and common) problem. You may not be able to complete remove stress from your life but make an effort to reduce your stress by reducing your workload, taking time for yourself, and by trying meditation or yoga.

Chapter Three: Men's Digestive Health

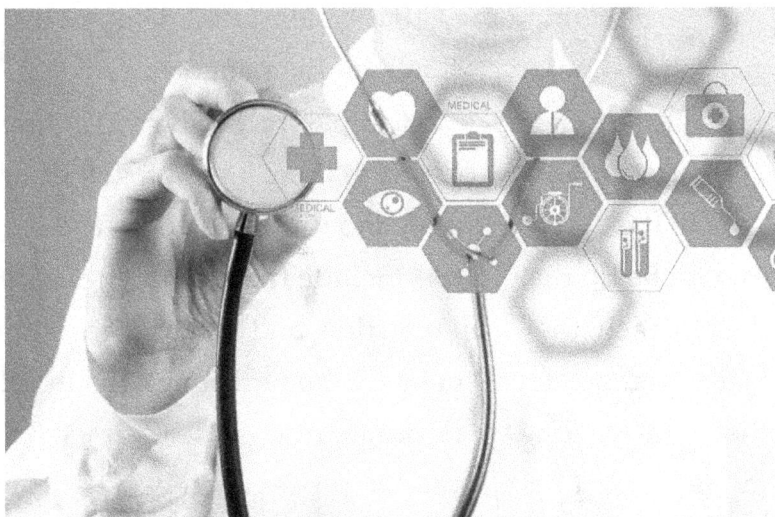

Your body is a well-oiled machine made up of different systems – if one of them is not running properly, it can throw everything out of whack. This is particularly true for the digestive system. If your digestive system isn't working well, you may not be able to absorb nutrients efficiently and that can affect your energy level, your concentration, and your overall health. In this chapter you will learn the basics about some of the most common digestive health issues affecting men as well as some simple tips to maintain good digestive health.

1.) Overview of the Digestive System

The human digestive system is made up of the gastrointestinal tract, the liver, the pancreas, and the gallbladder. The gastrointestinal tract (GI tract) is composed of a series of hollow organs that are joined together in a long tube that extends from the mouth to the anus. The organs that make up the GI tract include the mouth, the esophagus, the stomach, the small intestine, and the large intestine. When you eat, food enters the body through the mouth and then passes along to the anus through the GI tract. Bacteria in the GI tract help to aid the process of digestion as well.

In addition to the hollow organs that make up the GI tract, there are also several solid organs that are included in the digestive system. The pancreas produces digestive enzymes into the intestines to help facilitate digestion and hormones that are secreted into the bloodstream. The liver receives nutrients in blood from capillaries that absorb the nutrients through the wall of the intestines. The blood is then processed to remove bacteria and foreign particles and to further break down nutrients for use throughout the body. The gallbladder helps to rid the body of waste products through the secretion of bile and it helps with the absorption of fats.

The process of digestion is how food is broken down into nutrients which the body then uses for energy, cell repair, and growth. The food must be broken down into smaller molecules that can then be absorbed into the blood and transported throughout the body by the cardiovascular system. The nutrients into which food particles are broken down include carbohydrates, protein, fats, and vitamins. Each of these nutrients plays a different role and provides a different type of nutrition.

2.) The Top Men's Digestive Health Issues

Digestive disorders come in all shapes and sizes and they can affect both men and women. According to a recent study conducted by the Dallas VA Medical Center, an estimated 25% of adults suffer pain and discomfort related to digestive issues. Three of the most common digestive issues which tend to affect men more frequently than women include:

- Acid Reflux
- Ulcers
- Constipation

These digestive problems are generally temporary and can be relieved without any extreme treatments. There are, however, some digestive disorders which are more serious and may require special treatment. <u>These may</u> <u>include the following</u>:

- Gallstones
- Celiac Disease
- Gastroesophageal Reflux Disease
- Crohn's Disease
- Ulcerative Colitis
- Irritable Bowel Syndrome
- Diverticulitis

In the following pages you will receive an overview of each of these digestive conditions including their symptoms and various risk factors. Though some digestive disorders cannot be prevented, educating yourself about them can help to protect you.

a.) Acid Reflux

Acid reflux is the result of stomach acid flowing back up into the esophagus which can cause a painful burning under the breastbone. You may also develop a sour taste in your mouth and, in some cases, regurgitation. Acid reflux is also known as heartburn and it occurs when the sphincter (the muscle separating the stomach from the esophagus) becomes weakened so that it doesn't stay closed or it opens at the wrong time. Eating greasy or spicy foods can aggravate acid reflux, as can chocolate, caffeine, and alcohol consumption.

b.) Ulcers

An ulcer is a painful sore that forms in the stomach or in the duodenum (the upper portion of the small intestine). Anyone can develop ulcers, but they seem to occur twice as often in men than in women. Ulcers are caused by a certain type of bacteria and, if left untreated, it can cause stomach acid and other digestive juices to wear a hole in the lining of your stomach, causing excruciating pain that requires both hospitalization and surgical repair. Prescription drugs can be used to heal ulcers, though the process is very slow.

c.) Constipation

Like heartburn, constipation can affect both sexes but it seems to affect men more frequently than women. Constipation is often caused by a lack of fiber in the diet, though it may also be due to stress, the side effects of certain medications, or a lack of physical activity. Laxatives and stool softeners can be used to treat constipation but you should also make an effort to include more fiber in your diet. Exercising and drinking water will help as well.

d.) Gallstones

A gallstone is a hard deposit that forms in the gallbladder – the small, pear-shaped sac that is responsible for storing and secreting bile. According to the National Institute of Diabetes and Digestive and Kidney Diseases (NIDDK), more than twenty million Americans suffer from gallstones. These stones can develop if your cholesterol is too high or if your gallbladder doesn't empty properly. Symptoms of gallstones include a sharp pain in the upper-right portion of the abdomen.

e.) Celiac Disease

Celiac disease is an autoimmune condition in which the body's immune system begins to attack healthy cells and tissues in the digestive tract in response to the consumption of gluten. This disease affects approximately 1 in 133 Americans but many people who have it do not know it or they have been misdiagnosed with another condition. Symptoms of celiac disease may include digestive symptoms like bloating, diarrhea, vomiting, and abdominal pain as well as other symptoms like fatigue, depression, anemia, and even seizures.

f.) Gastroesophageal Reflux Disease (GERD)

Heartburn is very common and many people experience it once a week or more. If you have heartburn more than twice a week, however, it could be a sign of gastroesophageal reflux disease, or GERD. This is a chronic digestive disorder that affects as many as 20% of Americans and it can lead to esophageal cancer in some individuals, if left untreated. You should see your doctor if you have persistent heartburn, tooth enamel erosion, bad breath, pain in the chest or upper abdomen, nausea, or trouble swallowing or breathing.

g.) Crohn's Disease

Technically, Crohn's disease belongs to a group of digestive disorders classified under the title Inflammatory Bowel Disease (IBD). This disease in particular usually affects the end of the small intestine (called the ileum), though it can really affect any part of it. Crohn's is an autoimmune disease and a chronic condition, like Celiac disease, which caused the body to attack healthy cells and tissues in response to eating certain foods. The Crohn's and Colitis Foundation of America estimates that 700,000 people are affected by this disease. Treatment for this condition varies depending on the type and severity of symptoms, though it may include taking pain-relieving medications, immunosuppressant drugs, even surgery.

h.) Ulcerative Colitis

Another type of inflammatory bowel disease, ulcerative colitis also affects an estimated 700,000 Americans. Ulcerative colitis presents with symptoms very similar to Crohn's disease and it too is caused by the immune system mistakenly attacking healthy cells and tissues. The main difference is in the part of the digestive tract that is affected by the disease – ulcerative colitis targets the large intestine, also known as the colon. Treatment for this disease may involve dietary restrictions, anti-inflammatory medications, or (in severe cases) surgery to remove the colon.

i.) Irritable Bowel Syndrome

Frequent stomach pain or discomfort occurring at least three times a month for several consecutive months is often a sign of irritable bowel syndrome (IBS). This condition affects between 10% and 15% of the American population and it can cause symptoms including loose or watery stools, bloating, constipation, or frequent changes in the frequency and composition of bowel movements. The cause of IBS is unknown but it can be triggered by stress, eating certain foods, and by an imbalance of bacteria in the digestive tract.

j.) Diverticulitis

This condition is very common in older adults and it generally doesn't present with any obvious symptoms. It occurs when small pouched called diverticula form in weak spots in the lining of the digestive tract. These pouches don't usually cause problems but if they bleed or become inflamed, it causes diverticulitis. Symptoms may include fever, abdominal pain, and rectal bleeding and treatment usually involves antibiotic medications and a liquid diet to allow the colon time to heal. Severe or frequent attacks of diverticulitis may necessitate the surgical removal of the diseased part of the colon.

3.) Tips for Improving/Maintaining Digestive Health

Many people take their digestive system for granted. They eat what they like without giving any thought to how it might affect their digestion and their body as a whole. <u>If you are serious about keeping your digestive system (and your body) in good health, consider implementing some of the following digestive health tips</u>:

- **Focus on fresh, whole foods**. Everything you put into your body has an effect on your health – this is especially true for food. The more fresh, whole foods you eat, the less energy your body has to waste digesting processed foods. Whole foods are nutrient-dense and full of healthy enzymes which will help with digestion.

- **Chew your food carefully**. Do not rush the process of eating! The more thoroughly you chew your food, the easier it will be for your body to digest. This doesn't just have to do with physically breaking up the food – chewing also stimulates the production of saliva and digestive enzymes which also help with food breakdown.

- **Get plenty of fiber**. Having enough fiber in your diet is essential for healthy digestion. Fiber is what gives your stools bulk, making them easier to pass and preventing constipation. Adequate fiber intake can also prevent digestive disorders like diverticulitis and irritable bowel syndrome.

- **Be sure to include probiotics**. Probiotics are simply beneficial bacteria that help to facilitate healthy digestion. You can find probiotics in cultured yogurt, fermented foods, and even probiotic supplements made with live cultures.

- **Follow a regular eating schedule**. The body is like a well-oiled machine and it runs best on a schedule. To improve your digestive health, try to eat small meals and snacks every few hours throughout the day – avoid eating very large meals if you can.

- **Get some daily exercise**. In simple terms, regular exercise helps to keep things moving. Regular exercise can not only improve your health in general but it also helps to move food through your digestive system, preventing constipation.

- **Drink plenty of water**. Proper hydration is extremely important for healthy digestion. Things like coffee and soda can dehydrate your body, so limit your consumption of these beverages and drink plenty of water – aim for eight 8-ounce glasses a day.

- **Reduce your consumption of fats**. Foods that are high in fat can put extra stress on your digestive system, slowing everything down and increasing your risk for constipation. Don't avoid fat completely, but focus on healthy fats like monounsaturated fats and omega fatty acids.

Chapter Four: Men's Respiratory Health

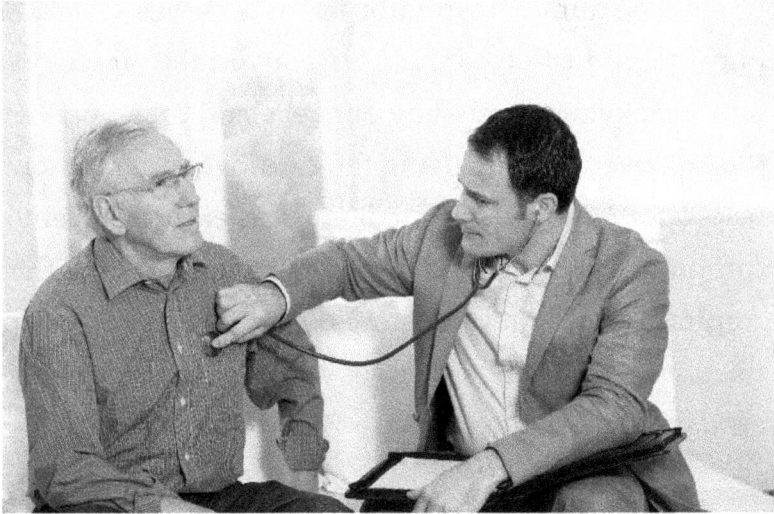

Breathing is an automatic function and one we often take for granted. You may not realize how nice it is to be able to breathe deeply and regularly until your breathing becomes impaired. Lung health is not something you should take for granted and there are many simple things you can do to improve and maintain good respiratory health. In this chapter you will receive some background information about the respiratory system and common respiratory health issues. You will also receive some helpful tips for improving your respiratory health.

1.) Overview of the Respiratory System

The human respiratory system serves several important functions. It helps to convert the air we breathe into the oxygen needed by our cells and transports it throughout the body using the cardiovascular system. The respiratory system also facilitates gas exchange, removing carbon dioxide from the body. The main organ of the respiratory system is the lungs – they are like giant sponges filled with thousands of tubes and tiny air sacs where the exchange of oxygen and carbon dioxide occurs.

Aside from the lungs, there are several other parts of the respiratory system - namely the nose and the trachea. As you breathe, air enters the body through the nose and it passes through the sinuses – hollow spaces in the skull which help to regulate the temperature and humidity of the air you breathe. The trachea filters the air you breathe, allowing it to flow into the bronchi, two tubes that then carry the air into the lungs. The bronchi are lined with tiny hairs called cilia which are covered in mucus that collects the dust, germs, and other airborne particles you breathe so they don't travel to the lungs.

The bronchial tubes transport air from the trachea into the two lobes of the lungs. The right side of the lungs has three lobes and the left side has two. Each lobe is filled with tiny, spongy sacs called alveoli – this is where the oxygen-carbon dioxide exchange takes place. The walls of the alveoli are incredibly thin, composed of a single layer of epithelial cells and very small vessels called pulmonary capillaries. As the blood passes through these capillaries, the oxygen is separated from the carbon dioxide – the oxygen is transported to the cells that need it and the carbon dioxide is exhaled from the body.

2.) The Top Respiratory Health Issues

The Office of Disease Prevention and Health Promotion (ODPHP) states that more than 23 million people suffer from asthma, nearly 14 million adult have COPD, and annual healthcare expenditures for respiratory issues total more than 20 billion dollars each year. While asthma and COPD are two of the most common respiratory disorders, other emerging respiratory issues include known to affect men include the following:

- Chronic Bronchitis
- Emphysema
- Pneumonia
- Lung Cancer

Disorders affecting the respiratory system can generally be divided into four categories. Obstructive conditions include things like emphysema and bronchitis while restrictive conditions include things like fibrosis, sarcoidosis, and pleural effusion. Vascular diseases include pulmonary edema, pulmonary embolism, and pulmonary hypertension, while infections and environmental diseases include pneumonia tuberculosis, and asbestosis.

In the following pages you will receive an overview of six of the most common respiratory health issues including their symptoms, risk factors, and popular treatment options. Unfortunately, some respiratory issues have a genetic component so you may not be able to avoid developing some of these diseases but you can take healthy steps to manage your condition.

a.) Asthma

Asthma is a type of chronic inflammatory disease that affects the airways, causing symptoms such as wheezing, coughing, chest tightness, and shortness of breath. This condition is caused by a combination of various genetic and environmental factors and it causes the tubes in the lungs to narrow, making it difficult for the individual to breathe – instances like this are called asthma attacks. In addition to the narrowing of the tubes, an asthma attack may also cause swelling to occur as well as mucus buildup in the airway.

Asthma attacks can vary in severity. For people who have only just started experiencing these attacks, they can be quite frightening and panic only causes the attack to get worse. Experienced asthma sufferers know that remaining calm is the best way to mitigate the symptoms, making the attack go away. The harder you try to breathe during an attack, the harder it becomes – you may even feel as though you are drowning. Common treatment for asthma usually involves an inhaled corticosteroid.

b.) Chronic Obstructive Pulmonary Disease (COPD)

Frequently shortened to COPD, chronic obstructive pulmonary disease includes both chronic obstructive bronchitis and emphysema. It is a chronic lung condition that makes it hard for the sufferer to breathe and it is becoming increasingly more common. In fact, COPD has become the third leading cause of death in the United States, affecting millions of Americans each year. Fortunately, COPD is both preventable and treatable.

The cause of COPD is generally long-term exposure to inhaled irritants such as cigarette smoke. Chronic obstructive bronchitis involves the inflammation of the lining of the bronchial tubes and it results in a productive daily cough as well as mucus production. Emphysema is a condition in which the alveoli in the lungs are destroyed due to repeated exposure to inhaled irritants. COPD may produce symptoms such as wheezing, chest tightness, shortness of breath, chronic cough, frequent respiratory infections, and lack of energy.

Approximately 20% to 30% of chronic smokers develop COPD during their lifetime, but it can also be caused by secondhand smoke, air pollution, or exposure to dangerous smoke, fumes, or dust in the workplace. This condition generally develops slowly, with most people being aged 40 or older when they start showing signs of the disease. People with COPD have an increased risk for heart disease, lung cancer, high blood pressure, and even depression. Treatment usually involves various medications to help relax the muscles constricting the airway and to decrease inflammation.

c.) Chronic Bronchitis

There are two types of bronchitis – acute and chronic. Acute bronchitis frequently accompanies an acute viral illness like influenza or cold and it is characterized by the development of a cough or a sensation in the back of the throat. Chronic bronchitis is a type of chronic obstructive pulmonary disease (COPD) which is characterized by a productive cough that lasts for at least three months. In addition to cough, symptoms of chronic bronchitis may include fatigue, chest tightness or discomfort, shortness of breath, chills, fever, and mucus production.

d.) Emphysema

Emphysema is a condition characterized by the gradual and progressive damage of lung tissue, particularly the thinning and destruction of the alveoli in the lungs. The main cause of emphysema is cigarette smoking, though it can also develop in people exposed to a great deal of secondhand smoke over a number of years. Along with chronic bronchitis, emphysema is one of the two main diseases that makes up chronic obstructive pulmonary disease (COPD) and it is not curable, though it can be managed with various treatments.

e.) Pneumonia

Pneumonia is a type of infection that causes inflammation of the alveoli (air sacs) in the lungs, causing them to fill with fluid or pus which can cause difficulty breathing. This infection can be caused by various types of bacteria, viruses, or fungi and, in addition to difficulty breathing, it may also cause cough, fever, and chills. The seriousness of this infection can vary, though it tends to be most dangerous for infants and for people over the age of 65 as well as for individuals with weakened immune systems or other health problems. There is no cure for this disease, though various treatments may help to improve quality of life and reduce symptoms.

f.) Lung Cancer

According to the American Cancer Society, there are three main types of lung cancer, each with its own specified course of treatment and prognosis. The most common type of lung cancer (accounting for 85% of cases) is non-small cell lung cancer and subtypes include adenocarcinoma, large cell carcinoma, and squamous cell carcinoma. Small cell lung cancer accounts for 10% to 15% of cases and it is a fast-spreading type of lung cancer. Lung carcinoid tumors account for fewer than 5% of cases and they tend to grow slowly – they rarely spread.

The symptoms of lung cancer may vary depending on the type and the progression. Common symptoms of lung cancer include persistent cough, change in color of sputum, difficulty breathing and/or swallowing, hoarseness, harsh breathing sounds, chronic bronchitis or pneumonia, and coughing up blood. The treatment options for cancer vary as well, ranging from surgery for stage I and stage II cases to radiation treatments, chemotherapy, and various medications.

3.) Tips to Improve and Maintain Respiratory Health

The human body has a number of natural defenses in place, including those that help to filter dirt, dust, and germs out of the air you breathe so it doesn't get into your lungs. Unfortunately, many people develop habits that can damage their lungs or, at the very least, impair their respiratory health. <u>Below you will find an assortment of respiratory health tips</u>:

- **Don't smoke, or stop smoking**. The main cause of lung cancer is smoking, though you can develop lung cancer as a result of secondhand smoke as well. At the very least, smoking can cause chronic inflammation in your lungs which can lead to chronic bronchitis and COPD.

- **Avoid air pollution**. Depending where you live, you may not be able to avoid air pollution entirely but you can be smart about reducing your exposure to pollutants like cigarette smoke, dust, and mold.

- **Maintain good hygiene**. Washing your hands and avoiding contact with people who are sick are the most effective means of protecting yourself against respiratory infections – you should also make sure to get an annual flu shot.

- **Engage in regular physical activity**. Not only is regular exercise good for your cardiovascular health, but it can also increase your lung capacity. Even if you can't do any strenuous exercise, there are some moderate or low-impact exercises you can try – even simple breathing exercises can be beneficial!

- **Maintain a healthy bodyweight**. The more weight you carry around, the more stress it puts on your lungs and other bodily systems. Following a healthy diet and getting regular exercise are the best ways to achieve and maintain a healthy bodyweight.

- **Keep the air in your home clean**. Even if you can't avoid environmental pollutants where you live, you can keep the air in your home clean by installing a purification system or simply by using a dehumidifier. At the very least, make sure to replace the filter on your AC system once a month.

Chapter Five: Men's Mental Health

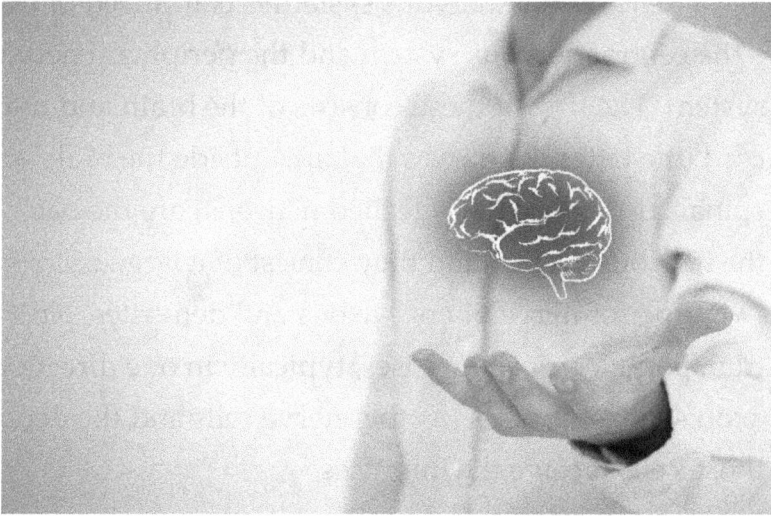

The term "mental health" refers to your overall psychological well-being. You may not be able to prevent mental illness if it is in your genes, but you do not have to become a slave to your illness – simply learning about your condition can empower you to take back control of your life. In this chapter you will find an overview of the brain and nervous system so you can better understand the effects of common mental health issues known to affect men. You will also receive some practical tips for improving and maintain both your mental and emotional health.

1.) Overview of the Brain and Nervous System

The human nervous system is comprised of two parts – the central nervous system and the peripheral nervous system. The first of these consists of the brain and the spinal cord, the latter the nerves that are outside the brain and spinal cord. Nerve cells (called neurons) are the basic unit of the nervous system and they consist of a large cell body and two types of nerve fibers – axons and dendrites. Nerves transport electrical impulses, typically in one direction – the axon sends impulses to other nerve cells and the dendrites of those cells receive the impulses.

The points at which nerve cells come into contact with each other are called synapses and the axons of the nerves secrete special chemical messengers called neurotransmitters. These chemicals trigger the receptors on the dendrites of the next nerve cell to produce an entirely new electrical current. Different types of neurotransmitters are used to transmit different impulses.

The central nervous system – the brain and spinal cord – consist of both gray and white matter. Gray matter is made up of nerve cells bodies, axons and dendrites, glial cells, and capillaries. White matter contains comparatively few cell bodies, consisting primarily of axons wrapped in multiple layers of myelin (this is what gives white matter its white color). The myelin protects the axons and it also speeds up the conduction of nerve impulses.

The number of connections nerve cells have with other nerve cells is constantly increasing and decreasing – this explains, in part, the way people are able to learn new things, adapt to changes, and form memories. The brain and spinal cord, however, rarely produce new nerve cells – this is why severe brain damage is typically irreversible. The exception to this rule is a part of the brain called the hippocampus which is where new memories are formed – it is also the part of the brain responsible for emotion.

The human brain consists of three main parts – the cerebrum, the brain stem, and the cerebellum. The cerebrum is the largest part of the brain and it consists of the cerebral cortex, white matter, and an assortment of subcortical structures. The cerebrum is divided into two halves, each of which contains various lobes. The frontal lobes are responsible for controlling motor skills, intellectual processes like speech and thought, and facial expressions – it is also responsible for coordinating expressions with moods and feelings.

The parietal lobe is responsible for interpreting sensory information, controlling body and limb position, influencing mathematical and language skills, and storing spatial memories. The occipital lobes process and interpret vision, form visual memories, and integrate visual perceptions with spatial information. The temporal lobes are responsible for generating memory and emotion, processing events into long-term memory, and comprehending sound and images.

The brain stem connects the cerebrum of the brain with the spinal cord and it contains a system of nerve cells and fibers. This system is what controls your level of consciousness and alertness – it also regulates critical bodily function like breathing, swallowing, heartbeat, and blood pressure. Consciousness is lost when the brain stem sustains severe damage and automatic functions may cease as well. Once this happens, death usually follows shortly thereafter. If the brain stem remains intact and damage is only sustained to the cerebrum, the body may still live even though movement and consciousness is impossible.

The cerebellum is the part of the brain that sits below the cerebrum, just above the brain stem, and it is responsible for coordinating bodily movements. The cerebellum receives information from the cerebral cortex about the positioning of the limbs and uses that information to help the limbs move accurately and smoothly by adjusting posture and muscle tone. The cerebellum also interacts with parts of the brain stem called vestibular nuclei which connect to the organs of balance located in the inner ear – these structures work together to create a sense of balance that allows you to walk upright. Your cerebellum also stores the memory of practiced movements which enables you to achieve highly coordinated movements with great speed and balance – an experienced ballet dancer's pirouette, for example.

2.) *The Top Men's Mental Health Issues*

According to the Kim Foundation, about 26% of Americans (more than 1 in 4) over the age of 18 suffer from some kind of diagnosable mental disorder. Furthermore, mental illness is the leading cause of disability in the U.S. for individuals aged 15 to 44. Mental illness issues can affect people of both sexes and of all ages and ethnicities. Even so, certain disorders and mental disturbances seem to affect men more frequently than women. For example, men are four times as likely as women to die by suicide and some conditions (like schizophrenia) tend to manifest earlier in men than in women.

It is unfortunate but true that there is a very strong stigma against mental illness in the United States. Many people still do not understand mental health issues and a staggering number do not believe that they are real, diagnosable diseases. These are just a few of the many reasons why a large percentage of people suffering from mental illness fail to seek treatment. Instead, they choose to suffer in silence and they often get worse, not better.

Again, mental illness can affect men just as much as women, but certain disorders seem to be more common in men than in women. <u>The most common mental health issues affecting men include the following</u>:

- Depression
- Bipolar Disorder
- Post-Traumatic Stress Disorder
- Social Anxiety Disorders
- Obsessive-Compulsive Disorder

In the following pages you will receive an overview of these five mental health issues including some basic background information about what these disorders are, how they manifest, and how they can be treated.

a.) Depression

It is estimated that as many as 6 million American men suffer from depression each year. What is interesting, however, is that an NIMH study revealed that many men suffering from depression symptoms were unaware that they were depressed – they did not make the connection between various physical symptoms (like headaches, digestive issues, and chronic pain) and their mental health. In many cases, men get caught up in concerns about masculinity and pride and, as a result, many fail to realize that they have a problem, let alone seek help.

Depression can manifest in different individuals in different ways. Some of the most common symptoms of depression include sad or depressed mood, feelings of guilt or hopelessness, loss of interest in things once enjoyed, change in appetite or energy, and/or suicidal thoughts. Depression ranges in severity from one individual to another and some treatments work best for some people but are ineffective for others. The two most common treatments for depression are anti-depressant medication and psychotherapy – a combination of the two is proven to be more effective than either option individually.

b.) Bipolar Disorder

At one time known as manic-depression, bipolar disorder is a form of mental illness characterized by swings between periods of depression and periods of mania. Mania ranges in severity from one person to another. In some people it remains fairly mild, inducing feelings of mild euphoria, increased energy and focus, spontaneity, and increased sex drive. In others, mania can become so extreme that the individual puts his own physical health at risk, engaging in dangerous behaviors or going on expensive spending sprees.

Bipolar disorder can be difficult to diagnose because many patients have a flawed understanding of the disease and therefore do not report their symptoms accurately. Many people assume that bipolar induces rapid mood swings from one end of the spectrum to another. While this may happen in a small percentage of cases, it is more often the case that episodes of depression or mania last for several days or weeks at a time. Psychotherapy is an effective treatment for bipolar disorder and there are a variety of medications which can be helpful. Most bipolar patients find that anti-depressants, however, are not effective – they have better results with antipsychotic medications.

c.) Post-Traumatic Stress Disorder

Often shortened to PTSD, post-traumatic stress disorder is brought about by the witnessing or experiencing of a violent, traumatic, or life-threatening event. This condition is particularly common in men who have served in combat and it can cause serious symptoms like flashbacks, paranoia, heightened vigilance, emotional numbness, even violent outbreaks, for some individuals. Some people suffering from PTSD eventually develop panic attacks and the condition can significantly impact their job, relationships, and quality of life.

Post-traumatic stress disorder can affect both men and women, but it sometimes affects the two sexes in different ways. For example, many women with PTSD feel anxious or on edge while men may take these feelings to the extreme, becoming angry or aggressive. Many men with PTSD also self-medicate with alcohol or drugs because they are ashamed or afraid to seek help. Unfortunately, PTSD sometimes leads to suicide.

d.) Social Anxiety Disorders

Many people who are extremely shy are actually suffering from a social anxiety disorder that causes severe anxiety in social situations. For some men, social anxiety disorder can become so debilitating that it interferes with their ability to go to work, to engage in social activities, or to maintain healthy relationships. What many people fail to realize about social anxiety disorder is that it is a diagnosable form of mental illness and it can be treated – you do not have to live the rest of your life in fear of being embarrassed in public or of meeting new people.

e.) Obsessive-Compulsive Disorder

Often shortened to OCD, obsessive-compulsive disorder is another form of mental illness that can become extremely debilitating. Men with this condition experience obsessions, compulsions, or both. An obsession is a repeated thought, urge, or mental image that causes stress and anxiety – an example is an extreme fear of germs or contamination. A compulsion is a repetitive behavior, often in response to an obsession – an example would be repeated handwashing.

It is normal to have little habits or quirks, but when your obsessions and compulsions start to take over your life, it can become a serious problem. Many people suffering from OCD feel as though they have no control over their thoughts and behaviors – they may feel powerless to combat them. When left untreated, OCD frequently gets worse and it can lead to serious disturbances and disabilities in terms of the ability to complete normal daily activities.

3. Tips to Improve Your Mental and Emotional Health

Your mental and emotional health includes not just your general mood – it also includes the way you feel about yourself, the amount of joy you derive from life, the quality of your relationships, and your ability to cope with difficulties and challenges. It is important to realize that good mental health doesn't require an absence of mental health issues – it is actually measured by your ability to deal with those challenges. Unfortunately, many people believe that mental health issues are something to be ashamed of and, rather than dealing with them, they deny their existence and, in doing so, make things worse.

You may not be able to prevent mental illness if you have a genetic predisposition for it, but there are some things you can do to prevent your illness from taking over your life. <u>Here are some general tips to improve your mental and emotional health</u>:

- **Make an effort to maintain relationships**. If you are suffering from depression or another mental illness, it can sometimes feel difficult (overwhelming, even) to motivate yourself to spend time with others. Maintaining relationships is important for your mental health, however, so try to engage in face-to-face interactions as much as you can.

- **Do things you enjoy**. Many mental health issues affect your enjoyment of things but you shouldn't give up on the things you love. Make an effort to take some time for yourself each day to do things you enjoy (even if you don't enjoy them in the moment). Sometimes you have to "fake it until you make it".

- **Get some exercise**. Not only can regular exercise have a significant impact on your physical health, but it can boost your mood and improve your mental health as well. The act of exercising stimulates the production of "feel good" hormones like serotonin in your brain.

- **Try to manage your stress**. Certain mental health issues can be caused or exacerbated by stress – various forms of anxiety are a good example. One of the best ways to minimize your mental health problems is to manage your stress. Make an effort to keep your work load manageable, take some time for yourself each day, and try to get enough sleep at night.

- **Follow a healthy diet**. Certain foods can have an impact on your mood and, in general, a healthy diet can help you to feel better both physically and mentally. Trans fats, sugary foods, refined carbs, fried foods, caffeine, and alcohol can have a negative effect on your mood. Fresh fruits, leafy greens, healthy fats, and lean protein, on the other hand, can boost your mood significantly.

- **Take time to help others**. Many people suffering from mental illness experience low self-esteem which makes it difficult for them to care for themselves. Even if you can't make yourself feel better, however, you may find that helping others boosts your mood. Try volunteering with a local charity or just be there for a friend in need.

- **Seek treatment**. The worst thing you can do for your mental and emotional health to deny the existence of a problem. If you are experiencing symptoms of mental illness, talk to your doctor. Your doctor will be able to help you determine the cause of your symptoms and to find the proper course of treatment that will relieve those symptoms.

Chapter Six: Men's Reproductive Health

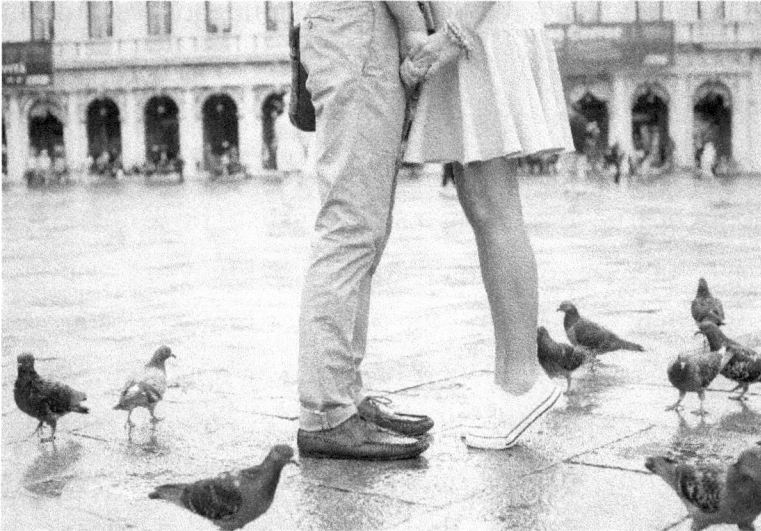

Many people mistakenly assume that reproductive health is a separate entity from overall health when, in reality, the two are closely linked. The reproductive system is linked to all of the other systems in the body so if it isn't working properly, it can lead to a breakdown in other systems. In this chapter you will learn the basics about the male reproductive system so you can better understand the effects of common male reproductive health issues. You will also receive some tips for improving fertility and for maintaining good reproductive health.

1.) Overview of the Reproductive System

The male reproductive system consists of several organs including the penis, scrotum, testes, spermatic ducts, and sex glands. The scrotum is a sac-like organ made up of skin and muscles which houses the testes – it consists of two pouches, each holding a single testis. The testes, also known as testicles, are the male gonads and they are responsible for producing sperm and the male hormone testosterone. Each testis is connected to a tube called an epididymis and the vas deferens is the tube which carries the sperm from the epididymis into the ejaculatory duct. This duct opens into the urethra, the tube that takes sperm (and urine) outside the male body.

In addition to the testicles, the male reproductive system also includes three sex glands which produce fluids that are mixed with sperm to make up the male ejaculate called semen. These three glands are the seminal vesicles, the prostate gland, and the bulbourethral glands – they are all located close to the bladder. The prostate gland sits just underneath the bladder and it is similar in size to a chestnut. The seminal vesicles are located posterior to the bladder and anterior to the rectum – they produce a liquid made up of protein and mucus which helps sperm survive in the acidic environment of the female vagina.

The penis is the external male sex organ which is located superior to the scrotum and inferior to the umbilicus. It has a roughly cylindrical shape and it contains the urethra, the external opening of which is located on the tip of the penis. The penis contains large pockets of erectile tissue which can fill with blood, making the penis become erect – this causes it to increase in size and to become turgid so it can enter and deliver semen into the vagina during sexual intercourse. The penis has the dual function of being the male reproductive organ and of allowing for the excretion of urine.

2.) The Top Men's Sexual Health Issues

Disorders affecting the male reproductive system are generally divided into two categories: penis disorders and testicular disorders. Both of these types of disorders can affect a man's sexual function as well as his fertility. Because the male reproductive organ is an external one, symptoms are usually obvious even in the early stages of disease. Even though these symptoms may be embarrassing, it is important to seek treatment promptly – most male reproductive disorders can be remedied when treated in the early stages.

There are a wide variety of different diseases and disorders which can affect the male reproductive system, but some of the most common are as follows:

- Priapism
- Peyronie's Disease
- Testicular Cancer
- Epididymitis
- Benign Prostatic Hypertrophy
- Testicular Torsion

In the following pages you will receive an overview of the most common male reproductive disorders including symptoms, causes, and treatment options. The more you know about these disorders the better you will be able to identify symptoms when they develop and the sooner you will be able to seek treatment.

a.) Priapism

This condition is characterized by a persistent, often painful erection that lasts for more than 4 hours. In many cases, the erection is not associated with any sexual activity and it is not relieved by an orgasm. This condition occurs when blood flows into the penis but it is not properly drained. Priapism can be caused by a number of things including drug or alcohol abuse, spinal cord problems, erectile dysfunction treatments, and certain medications including anti-depressants and blood pressure drugs.

Priapism is considered a medical emergency because if the erection continues it can cause scarring of the penis and may result in erectile dysfunction down the line. There are two common treatments for priapism. One involves draining the blood from the penis via a needle and the other involves medications which help to shrink the blood vessels, reducing blood flow to the penis. In very rare cases, surgery may be required to drain the blood and to avoid permanent damage to the penis. In cases where drug or alcohol abuse is a causative factor, treatment for the underlying condition is key to preventing the problem from recurring in the future.

b.) Peyronie's Disease

This condition is characterized by a plaque – a hard lump – forming on the penis. The lump can form on either the upper or lower side of the penis, typically in the layers that contain the erectile tissue. In many cases, the plaque starts with a localized are of swelling and irritation but it can eventually develop into a hardened scar which, over time, reduces the elasticity of the penis in the affected area. As such, Peyronie's disease can lead to painful erections as well as general pain.

Peyronie's disease can vary in severity from one case to another. In very mild cases where the condition does not progress beyond localized inflammation, the plaque may heal without treatment within 6 to 18 months. In more severe cases, however, the hardened plaque can reduce flexibility of the penis, forcing it to bend or arc during an erection, and the damage can be permanent. Treatment for this disease generally involves medical treatment to reduce the plaque or surgery to repair it.

c.) Testicular Cancer

Testicular cancer develops when abnormal cells inside the testicles begin to divide and start to grow uncontrolled. This type of cancer can affect children as well as adult men and it can develop in one or both testicles. It is also possible for a benign tumor to eventually become cancerous. Symptoms of testicular cancer usually include a lump, enlargement, or irregularity in the testicle as well as a feeling of heaviness or pulling in the scrotum. Some men also develop a dull ache in the groin.

The exact cause of testicular cancer is unknown, but there are certain risk factors which include an undescended testicle, a family history of testicular cancer, and race/ethnicity. Testicular cancer can develop at any age, but it most frequently affects men between the ages of 15 and 40. Treatment for testicular cancer depends on the progression of the disease and may include surgery to remove one or both testicles. Some cases may also require radiation and/or chemotherapy treatments. Testicular cancer is a fairly rare form of cancer but, fortunately, it is very treatable. Most individuals who develop testicular cancer recover completely with treatment.

d.) Epididymitis

The epididymis is the tube that wraps around each testicle and epididymitis is a condition characterized by inflammation of this tube. The epididymis helps to transfer and store sperm cells that are produced by the testicles – it connects the testicles to the vas deferens. Epididymitis can be caused by a number of sexually transmitted infections such as gonorrhea and chlamydia. In men over the age of 40, however, it is most commonly caused by a bacterial urinary tract infection.

Symptoms of epididymitis include pain and swelling in the scrotum, painful urination, discharge from the penis, and painful intercourse and/or ejaculation. This condition is generally treated with antibiotics and/or anti-inflammatory medications. The patient may also use ice to reduce swelling and a scrotal supporter to reduce pain. If the condition is caused by a sexually transmitted infection, the partner will need to be treated to prevent re-infection.

e.) Benign Prostatic Hypertrophy

Also known as benign prostatic hyperplasia (BPH), this condition is characterized by enlargement of the prostate. As the prostate becomes enlarged, it may restrict the flow of urine which can lead to symptoms such as difficulty initiating a urine stream, an interrupted or weak stream, incomplete bladder emptying, and straining. Though this condition can be unpleasant, it is generally not serious and it is very common – about half of all men over the age of 75 have an enlarged prostate. This condition can be treated with medication in mild cases and, in more severe cases, with surgery to remove part of the prostate.

f.) Testicular Torsion

Inside the scrotum, the two testes are connected by a structure known as the spermatic cord. If the cord becomes twisted around the testicle, blood flow may be cut off which can lead to sudden and severe pain as well as enlargement of the affected testicle. Testicular torsion is particularly common among men aged 25 and under and it often results from injury to the testicles or from strenuous activity – it sometimes happens for no discernible reason. This condition requires immediate treatment, usually surgical treatment, to prevent permanent damage.

3.) Tips for Improving and Maintaining Sexual Health

When it comes to reproductive health, one of the primary concerns is fertility. If you and your partner are trying to conceive a child, you should be concerned about your sperm count and your fertility in general. In regard to issues of infertility (defined as the absence of conception after one year of regular intercourse), men are responsible in about 40% of cases and low sperm count is one of the common reasons. <u>To help improve your sperm count, try some of these tips</u>:

- Avoid excessive alcohol use
- Do not smoke or do drugs
- Reduce exposure to environmental toxins like chemicals, radiation, and heavy metals
- Do not wear tight-fitting underwear
- Avoid sitting in hot baths or saunas
- Eat healthy, organic foods whenever possible
- Achieve and maintain a healthy weight

- Exercise regularly, ideally five times a week
- Take zinc and Vitamin C supplements

Another aspect of male reproductive health that you may be concerned about is your sexual performance. While performance is not directly related to fertility, certain reproductive disorders can affect your sexual performance. <u>Below you will find some tips to help you improve and maintain your desired level of performance</u>:

- **Take care of your heart**. When blood rushes into the erectile tissues in your penis, it causes an erection so your heart health is related to your sexual health. Issues with blood pressure and circulation can affect your performance so make take care of your heart.

- **Get some exercise**. Improving your cardiovascular health through regular exercise is a great way to improve your sexual performance – it can also boost your libido.

- **Eat certain foods**. Following a healthy diet in general is a good idea, but there are certain foods that can help increase blood flow – some examples include onions, garlic, bananas, peppers, avocado, pork, eggs, and olive oil.

- **Manage your stress levels**. Chronic stress can wreak havoc on your body, lowering your libido and increasing your blood pressure (this can affect your ability to achieve and maintain an erection). Psychological stress can also impact your ability to achieve orgasm.

- **Kick those bad habits**. Certain bad habits like smoking and excessive alcohol consumption and affect your sexual performance. Stimulants have been shown to narrow blood vessels and they have also been linked to impotence, so be careful about what you put into your body.

- **Get some sunshine**. Spending time in the sun helps to make sure you get enough Vitamin D but it also has an impact on your melatonin production. Melatonin is a hormone that helps to regulate sleep but it also reduces sexual urges – getting plenty of sun will help to keep your melatonin levels form getting too high and reducing your sexual desire.

- **Be careful about masturbating**. When it comes to masturbation, there is a fine line between just enough and too much. If you find that you don't have the kind of sexual stamina you want, masturbating may help to increase your longevity. Conversely, masturbating too often can make it difficult for you to last when you are with your partner.

Chapter Seven: Other Health Issues

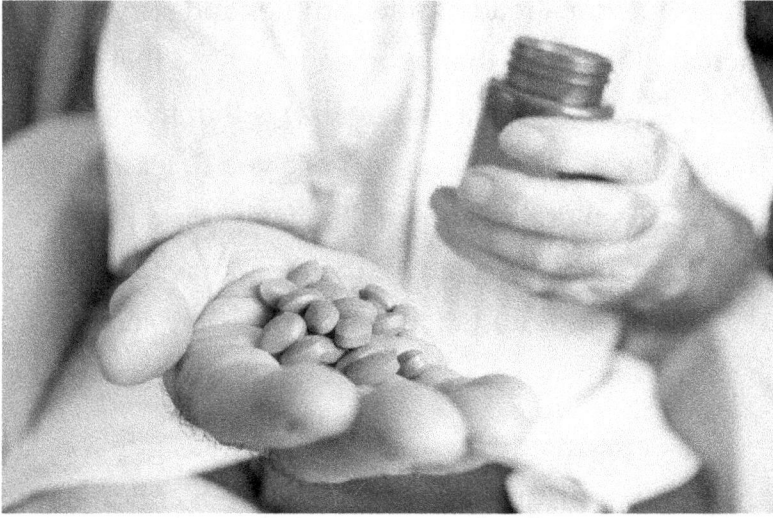

In addition to your cardiac, digestive, respiratory, and sexual health, there are some other aspects of your health and wellbeing that need to be tended to. In this chapter you will find an overview of common men's health issues in various categories including dental health, eye health, and sleep issues. You will also receive an overview of healthy weight suggestions that are catered specifically to men. Using the tips in this chapter you can round out your wellness efforts.

1.) Dental Health Tips for Men

As you already know, studies and surveys show that men are less likely than women to tend to their physical health – what you may not realize is that this also applies to dental health. It may also surprise you to learn that there is a link between oral health and longevity. Similar to routine physicals, men often ignore their annual or semi-annual dental checkups and that can lead to some serious dental health issues – primarily periodontal disease.

Periodontal disease, also known as gum disease, is the result of plaque buildup on the teeth and under the gums. Over time, this plaque hardens into a tough, porous substance known as tartar – tartar contains bacteria which produces acid that can irritate and even eat away at the gums. As the gums wear away, the bacteria spreads into periodontal pockets and it can even spread into the root of the tooth or the bones in the jaw, causing serious damage to the tooth and even death of the tooth.

This level of periodontal damage is generally irreversible – if things get that bad, the tooth must be removed. In the early stages, however, the inflammation of the gums is mild and can be reversed with daily flossing and brushing – this level of gum disease is known as gingivitis. Having regular teeth cleanings performed by a dental hygienist (on top of daily brushing and flossing) is the best way to prevent mild gingivitis from progressing into periodontitis, or severe gum inflammation, which can progress to tooth damage and bone loss.

Anyone can develop periodontal disease, but there are certain risk factors which can increase your risk. Smoking, for example, can not only increase your risk for periodontal disease but it can also make treatments less effective. Individuals with diabetes have a higher risk for developing infections, including gingivitis or periodontitis. Taking certain medications can reduce the saliva production in your mouth which can keep dangerous bacteria from being washed away, making your mouth more vulnerable to infection. It is also true that some people have a genetic predisposition toward oral health issues and periodontal disease.

The common signs of dental health issues include persistent bad breath, swollen or red gums, tender or bleeding gums, painful chewing, sensitive teeth, and receding gums. <u>Some of the best things you can do to preserve your dental health include the following</u>:

- Brush your teeth twice daily for two to three minutes using a fluoride toothpaste.

- Use a soft-bristled toothbrush and hold the brush at a 45-degree angle, positioning the head where the gums and teeth meet.
- Floss your teeth daily, gently inserting it between the teeth and using a back-and-forth motion.
- Replace your toothbrush every three months and after you have recovered from an illness.
- Visit your dentist at least once (ideally twice) a year for an oral exam and cleaning.

Maintaining good oral hygiene is not difficult – it just takes a few minutes each day and it is well worth the effort. It is particularly important for men between the ages of 55 and 90 years – this is when the risk for periodontal disease is the highest, though there is always a present risk if you don't care for your teeth properly.

2.) Eye Health Issues for Men

Just like your oral health, your eye health is easy to forget about when you are thinking about the top men's health issues. If you take a moment to think about it, however, you will realize just how important your eyes are – after all, you use them every day. Where would you be without them? Once you admit to yourself how important your eyes are, you have no choice but to admit the importance of eye health as well. Even seemingly minor eye health issues can lead to changes in your vision and could put you at risk for blindness.

To preserve your visual health you should keep up with annual eye exams – this is the best way to catch a problem in the early stages so you can get treatment and make a full recovery. <u>You should also take the time to familiarize yourself with common eye problems such as</u>:

- **Presbyopia** – A condition that develops when the lens of the eye loses flexibility – this is common with age and it can make it difficult for you to focus on objects up close.
- **Dry Eyes** – This condition may develop if your tear glands fail to produce enough tears. It can lead to itching and burning, though it rarely causes a loss of vision.

- **Cataracts** – A cataract is a cloudy area that develops within the lens of the eye. Cataracts are not painful and they may not affect your vision unless they enlarge or luxate (slip out of position).
- **Glaucoma** – This condition develops when pressure builds up inside the eye and it can lead to optic nerve damage if left untreated.
- **Conjunctivitis** – This is a condition in which the cornea of the eye becomes inflamed – it is sometimes called "pink eye" and it can cause redness, burning, itching, and tearing or discharge.

Medical or surgical treatment may be required if you develop one of the conditions listed above, though you will need to speak to your doctor for a diagnosis first. <u>In addition to keeping up with annual eye exams, here are some general tips to help preserve your eye health</u>:

- If you wear contact lenses, be sure to replace them as often as recommended and always clean them with fresh solution before putting them in.
- When spending extended time in front of a computer or television screen, give your eyes a periodic break using the 20-20-20- rule (every 20 minutes, focus on a spot 20 feet away for 20 seconds).
- Watch your caffeine intake – two servings of caffeinated beverages a day can actually be good for your eyes, but more than that may be detrimental.

- Keep some saline solution around the house just in case you get something in your eye – rinse it thoroughly with the saline solution for 10 to 15 minutes.
- Eat foods that are good for your eyes – this includes dark-colored berries, leafy greens and cold-water fish (for the omega-3 fatty acids).
- When you spend time outside in the sun, shield your eyes with sunglasses that offer 100% UVA and UVB protection.

If you experience any kind of problem with your vision or with your eyes, do not ignore it! Seek medical attention sooner rather than later – it is not worth risking your ability to see.

3.) Sleep Issues in Men

Though there is little definitive evidence, recent studies suggest that there are significant differences in sleep patterns between men and women. What is knowns, however, is that men are less likely than women to suffer from insomnia, but more likely to develop sleep apnea. It could also simply be the case that men may experience sleep apnea symptoms differently from women. According to the National Sleep Foundation, obstructive sleep apnea is frequently misdiagnosed in women compared to men – it is often mistaken for depression or hypertension.

While each individual has his own unique sleep habits and patterns, there are certain common signs that indicate you are not getting enough sleep – they include:

- Feeling tired or low in energy during the day
- Having a hard time focusing on work or school
- Feeling unmotivated or having trouble getting going
- Starting to doze off when not focused on an activity
- Feeling grouchy, irritable, or losing your temper

There are many reasons why you might not be getting the sleep you need. Sometimes there simply are not enough hours in the day to fulfil your work and family obligations in addition to getting a full night's sleep. Even if you do have enough time to get a full night's sleep, the quality of your sleep might still be poor. Stress, significant life changes, dietary habits, and lifestyle changes can all impact your quality of sleep. Certain medical conditions like asthma, arthritis, heart disease, and epilepsy could even be preventing you from sleeping well.

Sleep disorders can affect both men and women but some of the disorders that tend to affect men more frequently include obstructive sleep apnea, narcolepsy, and delayed sleep phase disorder. Obstructive sleep apnea is a condition in which you experience pauses in breathing while asleep – this can happen just a few times each night or hundreds of times per night. Even if you do not become fully conscious, these pauses in breathing wake you up and interrupt your sleep, causing you to feel unrested in the morning, even if you were in bed for 8 hours.

Narcolepsy is a condition which causes you to suddenly fall asleep, often while engaging in normal daily activities like walking, eating, or driving. This condition typically develops in men between the ages of 12 and 20 and it can stay with you for the duration of your life – it will not get better without some kind of treatment. Medications are usually effective in treating narcolepsy and in helping you to achieve a normal sleep pattern. Delayed sleep phase disorder (DSP) occurs when you get into the habit of going to bed very late and it can make it difficult for you to fall asleep during normal sleep hours – you may also have a hard time waking in the morning.

Though certain sleep conditions require medical treatment, many sleep issues can be resolved by cultivating good sleep hygiene. Here are some general tips to improve your sleep hygiene:

1. Make an effort to go to bed and get up at the same times each day.
2. Give yourself a full 7 to 8 hours per day that is reserved for sleep.

3. Wind down about 30 minutes before sleep – turn off the TV, put away your phone or computer, and try to relax.

4. Keep your room dark and comfortable for sleep – use blackout curtains if necessary and, if needed, use something for white noise.

5. Avoid drinking too much caffeine, especially late in the afternoon when it could keep you from sleeping.

4.) Healthy Weight Loss for Men

No matter whether you are male or female, the formula for weight loss is the same. If you burn more calories than you consume on a regular basis, you will lose weight. It is important to note, however, that men tend to carry their extra weight differently than women do, and some weight loss strategies are more effective for men than for women. If you are really serious about losing weight, you may want to start counting your calories – this is the best way to ensure that you are eating enough to support your metabolism without eating so much that you won't lose weight.

In order to lose weight effectively (and in a healthy way), you should start by calculating your basal metabolic rate (BMR). This is the minimum number of calories your body needs on a daily basis in order to maintain essential processes like respiration and digestion. <u>To calculate your BMR, use the following formula</u>:

BMR (for men) = 66 + (6.23 x weight in lbs.) + (12.7 x height in inches) – (6.8 x age in years)

Once you have calculated your BMR you can then use it to determine how many calories your body burns each day according to your activity level. <u>To determine how many calories you can consume each day to maintain your current weight, use the Harris Benedict Formula and multiply your BMR by the correct activity factor</u>:

- For sedentary men (little to no exercise): BMR x 1.2
- For lightly active men (light exercise 1-3x per week): BMR x 1.375
- For moderately active men (moderate exercise 3-4x per week: BMR x 1.55
- For very active men (hard exercise 6-7x per week): BMR x 1.725
- For extra active men (very hard exercise and 2x daily training or a physical job): BMR x 1.9

After calculating your maintenance calories using the formulas provided, all you need to do is create a calorie deficit in order to lose weight. You can create a calorie deficit by reducing your calorie intake by a few hundred calories or by increasing your exercise. In addition to creating a calorie deficit you should consider adding some strength training to your routine. Muscle burns more calories than fat so increasing your lean muscle mass will send your metabolism into high gear, helping you to burn more calories on a daily basis.

Chapter Eight: Nutrition and Exercise

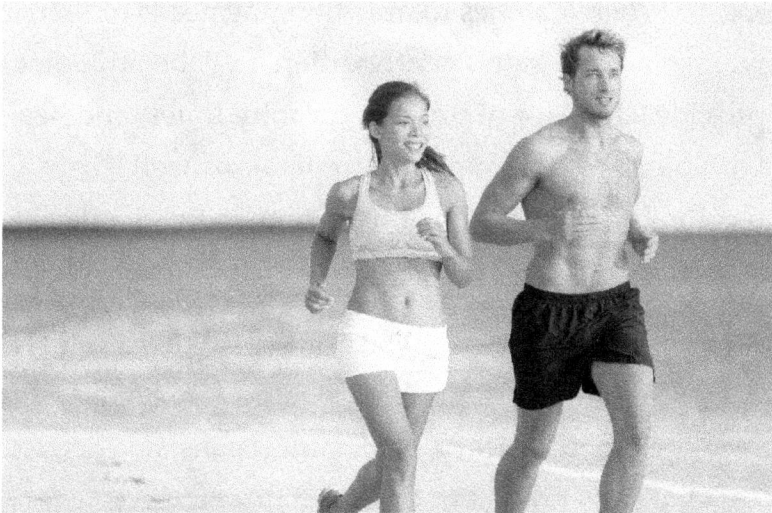

In addition to increasing your awareness of various men's health issues, you should also learn the basics of good nutrition and healthy exercise. If you've read through the whole book to this point, you will remember that healthy diet and exercise tips were on the list for all of the various health issues mentioned to this point. There is no denying the connection between a good diet, regular exercise, and general health and wellbeing. In this chapter you will find some general nutrition advice and some healthy exercise guidelines to follow.

1.) General Nutrition Advice for Men

When it comes to nutrition, the needs of men and women are not significantly different. A healthy diet should provide a balance of protein, carbohydrates, and healthy fats with plenty of vitamins and minerals as well. <u>Dietary recommendations change from time to time, but current recommendations provided by the USDA are as follows*</u>:

- 6 ounces grains (half should be whole grains)
- 5 ½ ounces of protein (include a mix of lean meat, seafood, poultry, eggs, nuts, beans, and seeds)
- 3 cups low-fat or fat-free dairy products
- 2 ½ cups veggies (variety of colorful veggies)
- 2 cups fruit (focus on whole fruits)

* These recommendations are based on a 2,000 calorie a day diet for an adult over the age of 18.

The guidelines provided above are just that – guidelines. You have some wiggle room when it comes to constructing a healthy diet. The important thing is to achieve a balance of nutrients and to consume mostly fresh, whole foods. Processed foods tend to be high in refined carbs and sugar, while being relatively low in nutrition. It is always better to eat foods that have been minimally altered by man. You do not necessarily need to switch to an organic diet, but you should seriously consider reducing your intake of processed food, fast food, fried foods, and sugary foods for your own good.

As an alternative to the dietary guidelines provided earlier by the USDA, you can also structure your diet based on certain macronutrient ratios. The term macronutrient simply refers to the three main nutrients – protein, carbohydrate and fat. The general recommendation for adult men is that at least 15% of the daily diet should come from protein – that is about 0.8 to 1 gram of protein per kilogram of bodyweight. If you are an athlete, your protein needs could be as high as 1.8g per kg bodyweight.

You may be surprised to hear this, but your recommended fat intake is higher than for protein – it is between 30% and 35%. If you are trying to lose weight, however, you should swap some of that fat for protein, reducing your intake to 20% to 25%. Remember, however, that your fat intake should come from healthy sources. Avoid trans fats and limit your consumption of saturated fats – monounsaturated fats are the healthiest fats. You should also get plenty of omega-3 fatty acids.

When it comes to carbohydrates, you need to be careful not just of how much you consume but also what you consume. Your total diet should be made up of 45% to 65% carbohydrates, but you should be focused on whole grains and low-glycemic carbs. Processed carbs are generally high on the glycemic index (GI) which means that they can cause your blood sugar level to spike and then crash – this is bad for your health in general and it can also increase your risk for diabetes. In addition to whole grains, other healthy sources of carbohydrate include fresh fruits and vegetables – they are also low GI.

In addition to watching what you eat, you should also be mindful of how much and how often you are eating. In order to keep your metabolism running at a steady rate, it is recommended that you eat several small meals and snacks throughout the day instead of just eating one or two large meals each day. Try to limit your portion sizes and eat slowly so you will feel when you are getting full and you can stop to avoid overeating. Eating too quickly can cause a delay in that feeling of fullness, leading you to consume more calories than you actually need.

2.) Exercise Guidelines for Men

The Centers for Disease Control and Prevention (CDC) recommends regular physical activity as a means of improving total health and fitness while also reducing your risk for chronic disease. The recommendations for adults is not as high as you might think – you should be aiming for about 2 ½ hours per week of moderate intensity aerobic activity as well as 2 days of strength training. If you engage in high-intensity exercise, the recommended amount you need will decrease proportionally.

Before you get too worried about these recommendations, wondering how you are going to fit it all in, remember that you don't necessarily need to exercise for an hour or more at a time. It is perfectly acceptable to break up your weekly workouts into 15-minute sessions. If you want the maximum benefit, aim for 30 minutes per day five days per week, but don't be afraid to break that into two 15-minute sessions each day. If you can fit in 15 minutes during your lunch break and another 15 minutes after work, that is completely fine!

Not only do you need to be mindful of how much physical activity you are getting, but you should also take care to get the right kind of exercise. Aerobic activity (also known as cardiovascular exercise, or cardio) is the type of exercise that causes you to breathe harder and makes your heart beat faster. If you aren't feeling challenged, then you aren't working hard enough! You don't need to push yourself to the limit, but you should be exercising at an intensity level that increases both your heart rate and your breathing for the maximum benefit. Here is a list of moderate-intensity aerobic activities:

- Walking quickly or uphill

- Performing water aerobics
- Riding a bike at moderate speed
- Playing doubles tennis
- Pushing a lawn mower

If you want to increase the intensity a little bit, try jogging instead of running, swimming laps, or playing an active sport like basketball. Another great way to maximize the cardiovascular benefits of exercise without committing too much time is to try High-Intensity Interval Training (HIIT). Don't worry – it sounds scarier than it is. HIIT simply involves alternating between periods of high-intensity exercise and rest. For example, you might jog at a brisk pace for 2 minutes then walk quickly for 1 minute before repeating the sequence.

There are plenty of different ways to engage in HIIT and you can customize a plan according to your physical capabilities and your fitness level. The basic idea is to maintain a ratio of 2:1 for exercise to rest. You can do HIIT with all kinds of activities, not just running! You can do it with swimming, biking, or even bodyweight exercises and you really only need to do it for about 15 minutes to experience the benefits. In fact, a recent study revealed that 2.5 hours of HIIT offered the same results as 10.5 hours of endurance training.

If HIIT doesn't sound like the right kind of exercise for you, you can certainly stick to more traditional options like running or walking. In the end, all that really matters is that you are staying active. You should also make an effort to include some strength training in your weekly routine. Strength training will help you to build lean muscle mass and muscle burns more calories than fat – this means that you'll be able to eat more calories without gaining weight. Just be sure to pair your strength training with a high-protein meal to maximize your gains.

Chapter Nine: Frequently Asked Questions

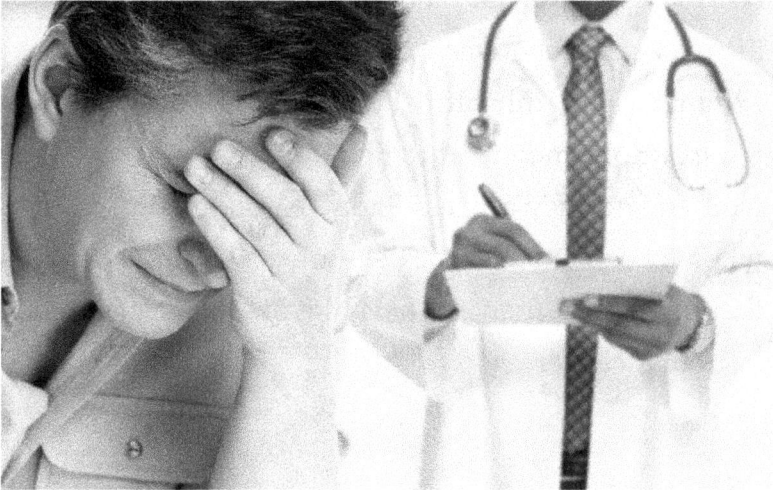

In reading this book you have received a wealth of information about general men's health issues as well as the specifics that apply to different bodily systems. There is no book, however, that is long enough to address every issue regarding men's health. This being the case, you may find that you still have some questions after finishing this book. In this chapter you will find a compilation of frequently asked questions about men's health issues to help round out your knowledge and understanding.

Q: *What are the primary factors affecting men's health versus women's health?*

A: Studies show that there is a measurable gap in average life expectancy between men and women – men also tend to exhibit certain unhealthy habits that can affect their health. For example, men tend to drink and smoke more than women and they are less likely to seek medical attention when a problem arises. There are also unique health issues that only affect men – things like prostate cancer and testicular cancer.

Q: *Why do men typically die younger than women?*

A: There are a number of health factors which come into play for determining lifespan and men face unique health challenges, especially as they get older. While men and women suffer from many of the same conditions, men often develop diseases earlier than women and they are less likely to seek treatment. Men are also less likely to keep up with annual physicals which is where many health problems are identified.

Q: *What are the best things I can do to maintain my health and to prevent chronic disease?*

A: The best thing you can do to maintain your health and to prevent chronic disease is to follow a healthy lifestyle. <u>Here are some simple things you can do to maintain your health for the long term</u>:

- Educate yourself about healthy lifestyle choices
- Follow a healthy diet
- Make an effort to exercise regularly
- Achieve and maintain a healthy weight
- See your doctor on a regular basis
- Stay up to date with your vaccinations
- Manage your stress levels
- Avoid smoking and drink in moderation
- Know your family medical history

Q: *What can I do if I don't have a doctor or health insurance?*

A: Just because you don't have a regular doctor doesn't mean that you have no options for healthcare. There are plenty of free and low-cost clinics out there, just contact your local health department for information.

Q: *Are there any health screenings I can perform on my own?*

A: If you don't have a regular doctor, you still shouldn't avoid routine health screenings – there are certain ones you can perform on your own at home. You can perform self-exams for your skin, mouth, and testicles.

Q: *What is my prostate and why is prostate health important?*

A: Your prostate is a walnut-sized gland made up of two lobes and it is located between the bladder and the rectum. The prostate is an important part of the male reproductive system and it can also affect your ability to urinate normally. Prostate problems can significantly impact your quality of life so do not delay in seeking treatment for prostate issues – it isn't worth it.

Q: *What is the difference between feeling "down" sometimes and being clinically depressed?*

A: It is completely natural to feel a little bit sad from time to time, especially if you are going through a difficult period in your life. There is a difference, however, between feeling down from time to time and being clinically depressed. Depression affects more than 6 million American men but it is still poorly understood, even by the people who have it. If you have symptoms of depression that last more than two weeks, the chances are that it isn't just sadness and you should consider seeing your doctor.

Q: *Are immunizations really necessary?*

A: There is a great deal of controversy regarding the risks of vaccinations for infants and children, but vaccines are not just for kids – they are important for adults as well. In fact, some doctors would agree that immunizations become even more important as you get older because your immune system may not be as strong as it once was. Your doctor will be able to tell you which immunizations are the most important ones for you to get but some of the most common vaccines are for flu, meningitis, and hepatitis.

Q: *What should I do if I think I've been exposed to an STD?*

A: It is very important to practice safe sex, but condoms do not offer 100% protection against STDs. If you think that you may have been exposed to an STD you should be screened for common STDs such as syphilis, chlamydia, and HIV. If you do not have a regular doctor, you can contact your local health department.

Q: *Where should I start with a regular exercise plan?*

A: Before you start an exercise plan, you should always check with your doctor to make sure you are healthy enough for exercise. Even if you have some kind of physical limitation or disability, there are always options and ways to customize an exercise plan to suit your abilities. If you haven't exercised before you should start off slowly and build up your endurance before you try any high-intensity forms of exercise.

Q: *What about alcohol? Is it good or bad for me?*

A: As is true for all things, alcohol is fine as long as you drink in moderation. Consuming one glass of red wine each day has been shown to reduce your risk for heart disease and moderate drinking may help to reduce your risk for stroke. Drinking to excess, however (especially on a regular basis), can be detrimental to your health. Any more than two drinks a day can lead to liver damage, high blood pressure, and various types of cancer.

Q: *Will my nutrition needs change as I age?*

A: Following a balanced diet is a must for men and women of all ages. It is important to eat foods from all five of the major food groups while limiting your intake of unhealthy fats and sugars. The USDA no longer recommends eating a specific number of servings from each food group every day. Rather, they now recommend eating all of these foods in proportion at each meal. Your plate should be divided into portions – the largest for vegetables, followed by grains, protein, fruits and dairy. As you get older, it becomes more important that you monitor your nutrition and you should watch your calorie intake as well.

Conclusion

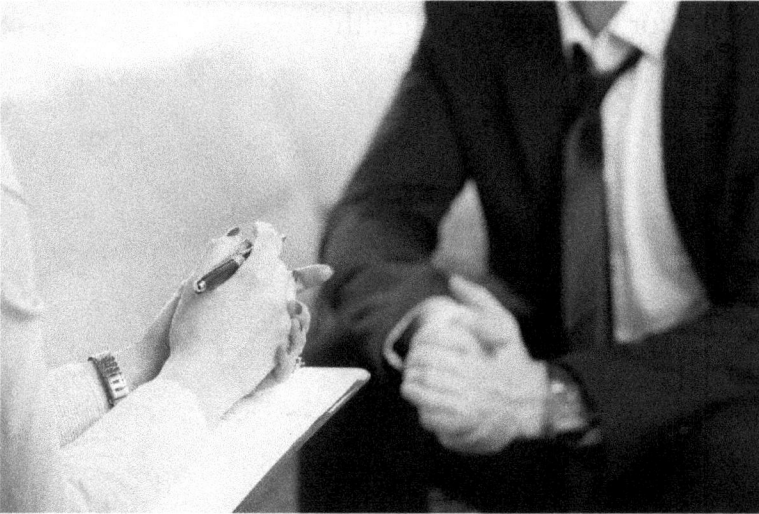

After reading this book you may be overwhelmed with information. After all, there are a great many ways in which your health can become compromised. Hopefully by now you understand the importance of keeping up with annual checkups, routine screenings, and yearly vaccinations. These things take a minimal amount of time but they can make a big difference for your health and wellbeing. Your health is not something you should be taking for granted!

So, if you are serious about maintaining your health for as long as you can, put the tips provided in this book to work in your life. You may be surprised to find how simple many of these tips are to incorporate into your life – you may also be surprised to see what a difference they can make for you and your health!

Index

E

F

G

H

M

N

O

Q

R

S

T

U

V

W

Y

References

"9 Ways to Improve Sexual Performance." Healthline.
 <http://www.healthline.com/health-slideshow/male-sexual-
 performance#1>

"A Glossary of Terms for Community Health Care and Services
 for Older Persons." World Health Organization.
 <http://www.who.int/kobe_centre/ageing/ahp_vol5_glossary.p
 df>

"BMI Calculator: Harris Benedict Equation." BMI-Calculator.net.
 <http://www.bmi-calculator.net/bmr-calculator/harris-
 benedict-equation/>

"Brain." Merck Manual. <http://www.merckmanuals.com/
 home/brain,-spinal-cord, -and-nerve-disorders/biology-of-the-
 nervous-system/brain>

"Common Eye Problems." WebMD. <http://www.webmd.com/
 eye-health/common-eye-problems?page=1>

"Health Checkups." Choosing Wisely.
 <http://www.choosingwisely.org/patient-resources/health-
 checkups/>

"How Much Physical Activity Do Adults Need?" CDC.
 <http://www.cdc.gov/physicalactivity/basics/adults/index.htm
 >

"Improving Mental and Emotional Health." HelpGuide.org.
 <http://www.helpguide.org/articles/emotional-
 health/improving-emotional-health.htm>

Kellow, Juliette. "Weight Loss for Men." Weight Loss Resource. <http://www.weightlossresources.co.uk/weight_loss/advice/tips-men.htm>

MacMillan, Amanda. "10 Tips for Better Heart Health." WebMD. <http://www.webmd.com/a-to-z-guides/prevention-15/heart-healthy/12-tips-for-better-heart-health>

"Male Reproductive System." Inner Body. <http://www.innerbody.com/image/repmov.html>

"Men: Stay Healthy at Any Age." Agency for Healthcare Research and Quality. <http://www.ahrq.gov/patients-consumers/patient-involvement/healthy-men/index.html>

"Men's Oral Health." Delta Dental. <https://www.deltadentalins.com/oral_health/mensOralHealth.html>

"Men's Top 5 Health Concerns." WebMD. <http://www.webmd.com/men/features/mens-top-5-health-concerns>

"MyPlate Daily Checklist." USDA. <https://www.choosemyplate.gov/sites/default/files/myplate/checklists/MyPlateDailyChecklist_2000cals_Age14plus.pdf>

Niemer, Ellen. "Nutrition Tips for Men." Alive.com. <http://www.alive.com/health/nutrition-tips-for-men/>

"Overview of the Cardiovascular System." Black Hawk College. <http://facweb.bhc.edu/academics/science/robertsk/biol101/heart.htm>

"Overview of the Nervous System." Merck Manual. <http://www.merckmanuals.com/home/brain,-spinal-cord,-

and-nerve-disorders/biology-of-the-nervous-system/overview-of-the-nervous-system>

"Pulmonary Disorders." Merck Manual. <http://www.merckmanuals.com/professional/pulmonary-disorders>

"Respiratory Disorder: Types, Symptoms & Treatment." Disabled World. <http://www.disabled-world.com/health/respiratory/>

Rona, Zoltan. "6 Ways to Boost Male Fertility Naturally." Alive.com. <http://www.alive.com/family/6-ways-to-boost-male-fertility-naturally/>

Santeramo, Elizabeth. "10 Top Health Risks for Men." Healthline. <http://www.healthline.com/health-slideshow/top-10-health-risks-for-men#1>

Sheehan, Jan. "Treating Digestive Troubles in Men." Everyday Health. <http://www.everydayhealth.com/mens-health/digestive-issues-in-men.aspx>

"Sleep and Men." UCLA Sleep Disorders Center. <http://sleepcenter.ucla.edu/sleep-and-men>

Spahr, Nancy. "Powerful Tips to Improve Your Digestive System's Health." Body Ecology. <http://bodyecology.com/articles/nancy_spahr_colon_therapist.php>

"Tips to Keep Your Lungs Healthy." American Lung Association. <http://www.lung.org/lung-health-and-diseases/protecting-your-lungs/?referrer=https://www.google.com/>

"Why is Life Expectancy Longer for Women than it is for Men?" Scientific American.

<http://www.scientificamerican.com/article/why-is-life-expectancy-lo/>

"Your Digestive System and How It Works." National Institute of Diabetes and Digestive and Kidney Diseases. <https://www.niddk.nih.gov/health-information/health-topics/Anatomy/your-digestive-system/Pages/anatomy.aspx>

Zimmerman, Kim Ann. "Respiratory System: Facts, Function and Diseases." LiveScience. <http://www.livescience.com/22616-respiratory-system.html>

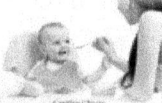

Feeding Baby
Cynthia Cherry
978-1941070000

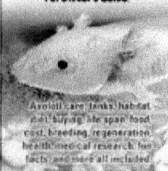

Axolotl
Lolly Brown
978-0989658430

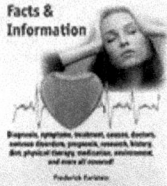

Dysautonomia, POTS
Syndrome
Frederick Earlstein
978-0989658485

Degenerative Disc
Disease Explained
Frederick Earlstein
978-0989658485

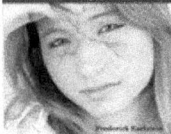

Sinusitis, Hay Fever,
Allergic Rhinitis Explained
Frederick Earlstein
978-1941070024

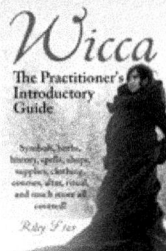

Wicca
Riley Star
978-1941070130

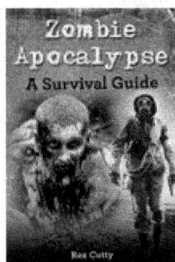

Zombie Apocalypse
Rex Cutty
978-1941070154

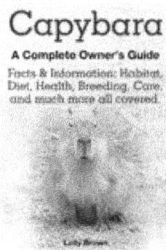

Capybara
Lolly Brown
978-1941070062

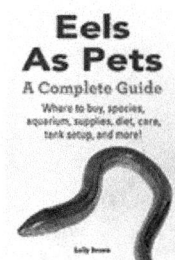

Eels As Pets
Lolly Brown
978-1941070167

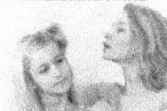

Scabies and Lice Explained
Frederick Earlstein
978-1941070017

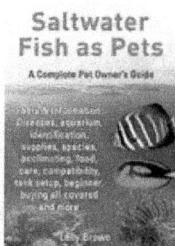

Saltwater Fish As Pets
Lolly Brown
978-0989658461

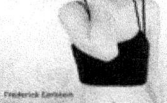

Torticollis Explained
Frederick Earlstein
978-1941070055

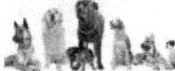

Kennel Cough
Lolly Brown
978-0989658409

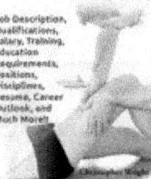

Physiotherapist, Physical
Therapist
Christopher Wright
978-0989658492

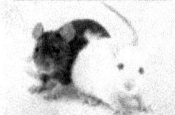

Rats, Mice, and Dormice
As Pets
Lolly Brown
978-1941070079

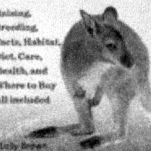

Wallaby and Wallaroo Care
Lolly Brown
978-1941070031

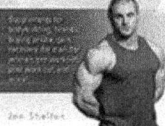

Bodybuilding Supplements
Explained
Jon Shelton
978-1941070239

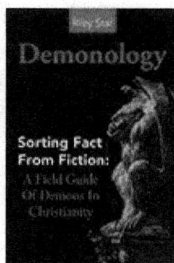

Demonology
Riley Star
978-19401070314

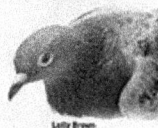

Pigeon Racing
Lolly Brown
978-1941070307

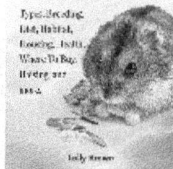

Dwarf Hamster
Lolly Brown
978-1941070390

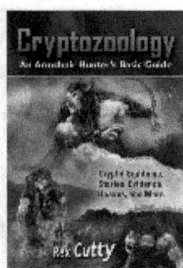

Cryptozoology
Rex Cutty
978-1941070406

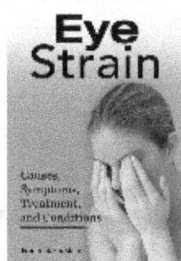

Eye Strain
Frederick Earlstein
978-1941070369

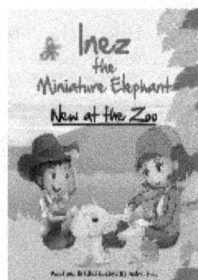

Inez The Miniature Elephant
Asher Ray
978-1941070353

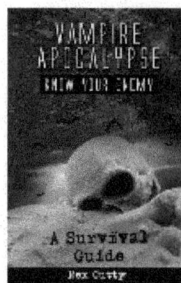

Vampire Apocalypse
Rex Cutty
978-1941070321

www.ingramcontent.com/pod-product-compliance
Lightning Source LLC
Chambersburg PA
CBHW050351280326
41933CB00010BA/1419